HOSPICE JOURNEYS
25 Memorable Stories

By Linda Hylan
Hospice Volunteer

Published by Angel Press 2018

First Edition: February 2018

Library of Congress Control Number: 2018903737

ISBN 978-1985877788

Hospice Journeys is a memoir of the personal experiences
of the author. Names and other details have been changed
to protect the privacy of the individuals portrayed.

Cover image: stained glass window in memory of the
author's brother

hylanhospicejourneys@gmail.com

CONTENTS

DEDICATION

This book is dedicated to two personal friends,

Bertha Dupree and Carol Maiello.

Through their courageous deaths,
they taught me how to live.

A SPECIAL THANK YOU

To my eldest daughter, Lori Hylan-Cho,
for her help in correcting tenses and grammar,

To my youngest daughter, Lisa Miller,
for her insightful comments honoring each
participant's final passing,

To my husband, Tim Hylan,
for his unflagging support throughout
this journey,

To my friend, Vickii Engel Thomas,
the catalyst in moving
Hospice Journeys forward, and

To Linda Johnson,
the angel who made this book
actually happen.

PROLOGUE

When I was in my late twenties, I read Elisabeth Kubler-Ross's book *On Death and Dying*. It was my first introduction to the concept of hospice. In the book, Dr. Ross talked about her own medical career and how she noticed that dying patients were the forgotten people. By focusing on the care of the dying, Dr. Ross gave them compassion and a voice. Although Cecily Saunders founded hospice in England, it was Dr. Ross who brought the Hospice movement to America. I knew when I finished reading her book that I wanted to become a hospice volunteer—someday. Someday, perhaps, when my children were grown and I had more free time. I promised this to God, saying "perhaps when I am in my fifties." I didn't consciously think of hospice after that.

In December 2000, my husband's work

transferred us from North Carolina to Maryland. Sometime in January 2001, I was driving around our new town while attempting to locate the post office. The directions I had been given weren't helping for the street I was on abruptly ended. As I sat in the car trying to guess whether to turn right or left, I noticed that the building directly across the street read "HOSPICE." I had an immediate flashback to my promise to God years earlier. Maybe I wasn't as lost as I thought. I drove into the hospice parking lot and went inside. I met with the volunteer coordinator who laughed when I told her about the coincidence of "being lost" and accidentally ending up at hospice. She said, "In hospice, we don't believe in coincidences, only 'God incidences'." And yes, she did help me find the post office!

I enrolled in the next hospice training session and graduated in May of 2001 at age 54. That's when I began visiting the wonderful people mentioned in this book. I began with a willing, compassionate heart but often, I tried to steer journeys instead of accompanying; I talked too much instead of listening and pushed too hard instead of allowing. However, the clients became my teachers. They were courageous, kind, strong, and forgiving.

I remember an incident that happened while I was still in volunteer training. At the time, I was grocery shopping at a local supermarket. As I returned to my car, a young woman stood nearby, holding her six-year-old son by the hand. She asked me what my license plate (GRAMALYN) meant. I told her my first name was Linda but that my grandchildren called me 'Grandma Lin.' The woman started to cry. It seems she had been very close to her deceased grandmother, and on this particular day, she had prayed for a sign from her grandmother. When she spotted my license plate, she felt it was the answer to her prayer as she had called her grandmother "Grandma Lane." These types of "coincidences" have continued to occur throughout my hospice calling.

With the exception of client names, which were changed in the interest of confidentiality, everything I have written in this book is true. Some stories include other-worldly happenings that were as surprising and inconceivable to me as I'm sure they will be to you. I've learned that dying can be an interactive process; one needn't be alone or in pain. I've learned that sharing and caring can make a difference, and that to be with someone when they are dying is both a privilege and a gift.

It is with deep gratitude that I thank all the participants who allowed me to share their end-of-life journeys.

Case #1

GETTING STARTED

Rick was my very first client. It had been three weeks since I'd graduated from hospice volunteer training and I was eager, but scared, to begin an assignment. I had preconceived notions about what it would be like sitting at a client's bedside, having him share his feelings about dying, and perhaps being the friend in need. We had been told to "meet the client where he's at," and not to bring our own agendas to the table, but this information seemed to evaporate when I went into the field.

Rick resided in the Alzheimer's wing of an assisted living facility, where the staff seemed warm and friendly. The nursing supervisor was giving out smiles, hugs, and encouraging words to staff and residents alike. She took me to the Alzheimer's lockdown unit and gave me the combination to the door lock. When I entered, a pet therapist was visiting patients with her three large Greyhounds. When I queried about Rick, a nurse pointed to a man sitting on a bench. He was watching other residents pet the dogs. He was wearing a sweat suit and socks, but no shoes. I asked where his room was, and the activity aide pointed to it.

I introduced myself to Rick but got no response. I took his hands in mine and helped him stand up. I then helped him to his room, with Rick shuffling forward while I walked backward holding onto his hands. I had brought my cassette recorder and some Chopin tapes with me, as I had been told he liked music. In retrospect, I realize I violated the first rule of volunteer conduct. Rick had been perfectly content watching the dogs. Why couldn't I have participated in that activity with him instead of taking him to his room?

When we reached his room, Rick immediately sat down on the bed. His Alzheimer's disease prevented a conversation. He definitely didn't understand who I was and kept yelling, "Whaddya want?" Luckily, the arrival of his lunch redirected his attention. The aide who brought the lunch put him into his wheelchair. I asked her if Rick could eat by himself, and she said yes. I assumed she meant he could feed himself—wrong! Rick just sat there like a stone. I asked if he wanted to be fed, and he said in a long drawn out fashion, "Alllllllllll right." He was very skinny and frail, not quite coming up to my chin. I looked at the food on the tray, which included meatloaf, potatoes, lima beans, applesauce, cottage cheese, and cake. I brought a spoonful of potatoes to his mouth; he opened for the food. I wasn't sure when to feed him the next bite, but suddenly he said in that drawn-out manner, "Allllllllll right." which appeared to be the signal to give him the next bite. Lunch took us nearly an hour because Rick ate everything! I remember thinking that if he died anytime soon, he'd definitely go to heaven with a full stomach. When he finished eating, he tried to get out of the wheelchair, so I asked if he was tired, and he said, "Allllllll right." I got an aide to assist him onto the bed, at which time he lay down on his back and fell asleep. I left.

After that initial contact, I visited Rick twice weekly for a few weeks. Mostly, we visited in his room because he spent most of his time lying on the bed. I think he recognized my face and the fact I would play taped Chopin piano music for him as he no longer said, "Whaddya want?" Also, I began bringing a folder of sheet music with me so that when I wasn't playing Chopin on the cassette recorder, I could sing some "oldies" a cappella. On one of these visits, a staff person asked if I would play the piano in the entry foyer so that other patients could also sing along. So, on my Monday visits when he felt up to it, I'd put Rick in his wheelchair, and together we'd go out into the main lobby. He'd sit next to the piano although he wasn't able to sing. I could tell he was listening and enjoying the music though, as his foot would tap to the beat.

On my Thursday visits, we'd stay in his room, and Rick would lie on the bed with his eyes closed. I'd notice that his eyelids would flutter whenever I sang "Always" or "In the Garden," so I included those two songs during each visit. Staying calm was a change for Rick because he was known in the facility as a screamer. He continuously yelled out his wife's name, which upset the staff and other patients. However, whenever I sang, he remained quiet.

Towards the end of his life, Rick couldn't get out of bed, so I visited him strictly in his room. It was luck that brought me to his bedside the afternoon of his death. The facility where he resided was holding a Saturday Open House when I stopped by with my sister-in-law to show her the amenities. While there, I entered Rick's room to check on him. His wife, one daughter, and a hospice social worker were sitting vigil at his bedside. I introduced myself to his wife, and she said she had been told that I brought music to Rick on my visits. She informed me that he had sung in a church choir all his life and that his favorite hymn had been "In the Garden." She also mentioned that he had played the ukulele and his favorite song to play was "Always." I then shared with her how he seemed to physically respond whenever I sang those two particular songs. She asked if I could sing to him while I was there. I bent over his left ear and quietly sang three verses of "In the Garden." I shared hugs with Rick's wife and daughter, and said my own personal goodbye to him. I thanked Rick for putting up with my inexperience and for helping me get through my first Hospice volunteer experience. I later learned he died that evening.

Case #2

WE AREN'T BUYING

My second hospice assignment, Anthony, was really half an assignment. My supervisor called to say there was another patient at the assisted living facility where I was seeing Client #1 (Rick).

Anthony already had a volunteer, but the volunteer was asking for reinforcements. Anthony and his wife of 67 years roomed together on the second floor. He was dying of prostate cancer, and his wife was talking about wanting to die at the same time he did. Everyone was concerned.

The first time I knocked on their door, Anthony's wife, Bertha, greeted me from an easy chair in the corner of their bedroom with a sweet "come in." I had been told that she had some dementia, so it didn't surprise me when she had trouble understanding who I was. She was gracious, however, and assumed from what I was saying and my hospice ID badge that I was there to help her husband. I stayed to talk to her for over an hour while Anthony slept through our visit.

Amazingly, as I was telling her about myself, we laughed at discovering we were both piano teachers. She had taught piano for over 50 years and could clearly recount many interesting stories about her students. I had brought my cassette recorder and a Chopin tape with me, so we sat and listened to the piano music together. She seemed to relax as the music played.

On my second visit, Bertha was sitting in a chair between her bed and her husband's bed, holding his hand. She continuously muttered, "Oh my, oh my" and occasionally would tell me stories of their wonderful life together, never letting go of his hand. From her musings, it was obvious that he had been the leader in the marriage, taking care of her all his life. Caretaking was a new role for Bertha. When her lunch arrived, I said I would leave so she could eat, but she begged me to eat her food as she said she wanted to die "when he did." I took a moment to explain how necessary it was that she remain healthy so she could keep Anthony's memory alive after he passed. We talked about how hard that would be, but how much Anthony would want her to live and enjoy the years she had left. I asked if she would like to listen to Chopin music while she ate, as I needed to go downstairs to visit my other client. She agreed and I showed her how to push the *eject* button when the first side of the cassette ended. Next, I showed her how to turn the tape over and hit the *play* button. As I was doing so, Anthony suddenly opened his eyes and bolted up to a sitting position on the bed. He glared at me sternly and in a very loud, authoritative voice said, "We're NOT buying!" Bertha burst out laughing, patted his hand and said, "Honey, she's not selling." With that, he lay back down and went to sleep. I've smiled many times over that incident.

I only knew Anthony two weeks before he passed away. Bertha grieved but decided to live. She joined our weekly sing-along sessions in the main lobby on Mondays. As serendipity would have it, our hospice paths crossed again six months later.

Case #3

SHE HEARD ME

Mabel was an edematous, bedridden elderly
lady who had been fiercely independent before
becoming sick. If you wanted to know how Mabel
felt about anything, all you had to do was ask! She
had end-stage emphysema with 24-hour oxygen
support, and also suffered from diabetes. The first
time we met, Mabel told me that she had been
born and brought up in New York State, and she
wouldn't go back to "that lousy weather if you paid
me a million dollars!" She was proud of the fact
that she had been a clothing merchant in New
York City in an era when women rarely worked
outside the home. She worked to support her son
after her husband died unexpectedly after 15 years
of marriage.

She said for the last few years she had been
living happily in Florida, but recently moved to

Maryland to be near her only son. Medical problems had forced her to enter the nursing home.
I explained to Mabel my role as a Hospice volunteer. I asked her how often she would like me to visit and how I could be of assistance to her. She said to come when I wanted and to read her a romance novel.

I brought a Nora Roberts novel on my next visit, thinking a mild contemporary novelist might interest Mabel. After reading a few chapters out loud to her, she announced in a loud voice that the story was "too boring." On my next visit, I brought a romance novel that had a bare-chested man clad in a loincloth on its cover. Mabel nodded her approval so I brought a chair up close to her bed on the left side for she was hard of hearing. It didn't help that she was tethered to a noisy oxygen machine on her right side. Mabel would make an occasional comment about the story, but mostly she listened quietly because the oxygen tubing made her mouth dry.

When I first started visiting, Mabel had been able to feed herself, albeit slowly, but after three weeks, she couldn't even do that. I remember the time I visited and politely asked how she was doing. She replied in her low, raspy voice, "I'm aggravated, very aggravated." Haltingly, she said that nursing home staff had been reduced over the weekend, and no one had time to help her eat, so she had spilled food all over herself, which disgusted her. I think she started to give up after that incident. When I asked what I could do to make things better for her, she surprised me by saying, "Bring me a root beer float!" I checked with the hospice nurse who said not to worry about the diabetes at this stage, so my visits to Mabel began to include stops at a local homemade ice cream store for either a root beer float or a malted milk shake. I would hold the straw to her lips, and as she drew the liquid up to her mouth, she would roll her eyes and say, "Heaven." I got tremendous joy out of seeing the way she relished those ice cream offerings.

I began visiting Mabel more often, and when I entered her room, Mabel would say, "Oh goody—treats!" I'd feed her some ice cream, read a few paragraphs of the Harlequin book aloud, and continue to alternate these activities until the ice cream was gone. I remember one embarrassing day when I realized that the couple in this romance novel was getting very passionate. I told Mabel that it looked like the lovebirds might have sex in the next chapter and did she want me to skip it? In an extremely loud raucous voice she responded, "Hell, no!" To her delight, I got up, closed the bedroom door that opened onto a public hallway, and loudly read the spicy chapter, replete with "quivering thighs and heaving bosoms."

My own cheeks got very red with embarrassment, but Mabel was pleased.

A month passed and I had gotten very attached to Mabel. One morning as I prepared to leave for the ice cream parlor on the way to see her, I received a phone call from my Hospice supervisor telling me that Mabel had passed away two hours earlier. I definitely wasn't ready for this news. I cried and sobbed for two hours. I remember yelling, "Damn it Mabel, we haven't finished the book yet!" Of course, it wasn't like I didn't know she was going to die—for goodness sake, I'm a hospice volunteer. By noon, I was all cried out and began talking to Mabel out loud. I told her I was sorry for my selfishness and that I knew she was in a better place and feeling well again. I asked her forgiveness but added, "We *are* going to finish the book." That night, I lit a candle and read three chapters out loud to her. My husband thought I had flipped my lid, but I felt like a woman on a mission. I continued this nightly routine until the book was finished, at which time I looked up and said, "I hope you heard me, Mabel." It was only then that my heart seemed ready to release her.

Ten days following her death, Mabel's son held a memorial service at the nursing home. During the service, I shared some of my fondest memories of Mabel with the attendees and thought our business together was finished. However, the following week, I received an e-mail from someone I had met during my hospice training who asked how my cases were going. I responded that my most recent client, Mabel, had died and that I had taken it badly. My e-mail friend said that we needed to get together for lunch as soon as possible, and I assumed it was because she wanted to console me.

A week later, I went to this woman's home for lunch. She surprised me by saying she was an intuitive and related to me that for the past two weeks, she had been hearing the name "Mabel" along with a three-word phrase. She had asked around but no one knew of a Mabel who had recently died, so she felt sure Mabel's message must be for me.

The three words truly brought me closure and an assurance that life continues after death. The words were "I heard her."

Case #4

DISCHARGED

I waited two months after Mabel died to accept my next client, Allen, who resided in a split-level house on a hill with a beautiful view. The house was owned by two nurses who had adapted it into a home for assisted living and nursing home patients. It provided a natural setting where clients received three home-cooked meals per day and individualized attention.

I recognized Allen immediately as the man I had noticed a month prior at a local nursing home facility when I was visiting another patient. At that time, he had been unresponsive and lay in a fetal position on his bed. Although he had been a biology professor for 30 years, Alzheimer's disease had caused him to revert to infantile behaviors.

In this more homey setting, Allen was still nonverbal, incontinent, and displaying rooting

behaviors with his mouth that sometimes led to
biting staff, but he wasn't in bed in a fetal position
anymore. Instead, he reclined in a lounge chair
facing a large picture window in the main room of
the house surrounded by other residents. I was
pleased to see the improvement in him physically.
I tried to find a modality in which to connect with
him on this visit. I talked in a soothing voice but
got no response. After an hour, I left.

On my second visit, I brought several cassette tapes of different musical genres to play, but
again, no response. I asked one of the nurses for
advice and she said that whenever she mentioned
anything about education or nature, he seemed to
listen and watch. I wondered if that would be the
connection.

I was pleased to find Allen improved on my
third visit. He was quietly chewing on a large
teething ring while seated in a Barcalounger in the
sunny main room. He was no longer pulling up his
knees to his chest. I had brought a horticulture
book with me and held up the pictures for him to
see. He stopped chewing and gazed at the photos
while I read the captions. At lunchtime, he ate his
lunch with very little assistance. This included
drinking three whole glasses of milk. It appeared
that the tender-loving care he was getting in this
new environment agreed with him.

I continued visiting Allen weekly, showing

him nature photographs each time. Allen surprised me one day when I was preparing to leave. He leaned forward for a kiss goodbye, which I planted on the top of his head. It wasn't long after this gesture that the hospice nurse determined that Allen was now too high-functioning to be under hospice care. Having a patient discharged from hospice *alive* was a surprise for me, but definitely a nice one.

Case #5

MUFFY

My fifth case was assigned shortly after Allen was discharged from hospice care. Her name was Myra, but she asked to be called by her nickname, Muffy. She was my first actual in-home patient. Her husband, Jim, met me at the door and took me to the family room where Muffy was lying on a couch watching television. I learned she was 54 years old, the same age as me, which made me think back to my original notion that most people in hospice care would be elderly. That idea was dispelled at my first Hospice training class when I learned that the average age of a hospice patient was between 40-60.

Muffy seemed upbeat but mentioned being overwhelmed by the number of hospice staff who had been visiting since she had been admitted to hospice care three days earlier. She told me about her pancreatic cancer, which had gone undiagnosed for eight months due to the "cavalier attitude" of her general practitioner, who had brushed off her symptoms as acid reflux. Due to stabbing pains in her side, she quit the job where she had worked for 30 years, and spent most of her days lying on the couch. Although her general practitioner eventually ran some additional tests, he claimed they were inconclusive, and Muffy continued to suffer.

After six months of being in pain, Muffy's husband insisted she seek a second opinion. The consulting doctor performed a CT scan and MRI, which revealed pancreatic cancer. Chemotherapy and radiation were performed but were ineffective. When the oncologist discovered that the cancer had invaded her liver, he suggested that Muffy enter hospice. As she shared this information matter-of-factly with me, I felt a deep sense of sadness for her situation. We chatted for another few minutes and then agreed that I'd stay in touch by phone rather than visit as Muffy was trying to regulate the number of people coming to the house.

When I called three days later, Muffy said that the Hospice nurse had been able to get her pain under control, which was a huge relief to her. She could now sleep for a few hours at a time, something she hadn't been able to do in months.

A week later, my next phone call was answered by Muffy's husband. He said she had slipped into a coma over the weekend and died Monday morning. I had a hard time mentally letting go of this case. I felt she had suffered pain unnecessarily due to an initial incorrect diagnosis. Too much time had elapsed before learning the truth of her condition, including that it was too late for any possible improvement.

Although I was grateful that Hospice was able to resolve Muffy's pain at the end of her life, I had to take a couple weeks off from volunteer work to resolve my own emotions surrounding these issues.

Case #6

BEST DRESSED

When I felt ready to return to active duty, I was assigned to a 78-year old woman named Valerie, who suffered from chronic obstructive pulmonary disease (COPD). Valerie lived in a first floor apartment with her second husband, Elton, who was her primary caregiver. It was evident from the moment I met him that Elton was very devoted to her. In fact, Valerie laughingly related that her daughter referred to him as "Saint Elton."

My first home visit was in October, a month after Valerie had been discharged from a lengthy hospital stay. She sat in a recliner with her legs propped up, wearing a nasal cannula with endless yards of tubing attached to an oxygen tank located in the hallway. She seemed a small figure in the chair, pillows on all sides keeping her secure, with her body leaning towards the end table that held her nebulizer. She weighed less than 90 pounds and her coccyx gave her a lot of pain, so she would list sideways to avoid aggravating it.

Valerie told me she had been born in Maryland but had spent over fifty years in New York State, which, coincidentally, was where I grew up. It reminded me of my hospice training in which an instructor had said, "There are no coincidences, only 'God incidences'."

With my first five cases, none of the clients had ever been willing to talk about death issues so it surprised me when, after five minutes of general conversation, Valerie began describing her casket and the complimentary clothing colors she wanted to be laid out in. She told me the casket lining was pink and she'd be wearing her brand new bluish gray Liz Claiborne suit, which should coordinate beautifully. Her husband sat on the couch across from us smiling and not interrupting. He seemed willing to let her express her end-of-life opinions as she desired. I felt an instant respect and admiration for them both.

I began visiting Valerie on Tuesdays and Thursdays for two hours at a time so that her husband could run various errands. Despite difficulty breathing, Valerie loved to talk. She told me her only offspring was a daughter who lived in Virginia. They were closely bonded and spoke nightly by phone. Valerie had always wanted more children but hadn't been "blessed in that way." She had been married almost 30 years when her first husband died; a few years after that, she married Elton, a widower. Valerie and Elton had recently celebrated their thirteenth wedding anniversary. Valerie spoke of her childhood and what wonderful parents she had. She remembered her mother only striking her once, and that was for "being sassy." I learned she had three sisters and one brother living nearby, and another brother living on the west coast.

As we got to know each other better on subsequent visits, Valerie would talk as if we had known each other all our lives. She fretted about loose ends: "How would Elton get everything boxed up after she died?"

She wondered who would go through everything and dispose of it according to her wishes. How would her sisters get along without her? Most importantly, she didn't want to "die over the holidays and ruin everything for family members." She said her dad had died in the month of December, which had ruined Christmas for the family, so she was thinking more about possibly dying in the spring! She said that although her body was to be laid out in Maryland, it would be shipped to New York State for burial. She hoped that the ground wouldn't be too frozen to dig a grave during the winter months. Even though she had a will in New

York State, one of her sisters told her it would not be honored in Maryland. Thankfully, this issue was eventually resolved so that she had a valid in-state will before she died.

It seems weekends were filled with out-of-town family who came to visit their small apartment. Valerie would tell me all about these visits when I'd see her each Tuesday. By mid-November, Valerie's 5-foot 8-inch frame had shrunk to 5 feet 4 inches, and her weight had dropped from 145 to 86 pounds, mainly due to the effect of Prednisone on her bones. A hospital bed had to be set up in her bedroom. It was positioned so that she could look directly down the hall and see anyone who entered the front door. I would sit on a kitchen chair brought close to the bed so I could hear her talk. Her voice had grown weak, but she continued to share whatever was on her mind.

On one of my visits, I brought her a white, handmade lightweight afghan she could use as a pretty coverlet to replace an old towel that sat atop the bed. Sometimes I'd find the afghan folded next to her as she "didn't want to get it dirty." Her next worry had become what she could "give me" because she so loved our visits. I explained many times that hospice volunteers were prohibited from accepting gifts of any kind, and that just knowing her was a gift to me, but she continued to fret.

By the end of November, Valerie had deteriorated considerably. One day as I sat next to her, she cocked her head to the side and asked what the voices were she heard. I listened but heard nothing. Another day, she looked towards the front door and asked about the man in plaid who had just entered. Although I saw no one, I got up and thoroughly checked the living room, dining room, and kitchen so I could reassure her. She then said he had ducked into the bathroom so I checked there also. This episode allowed us to talk about the "thinning of the veil" that separates us from the Other Side, and how she was the lucky one who got to glimpse or hear the Other Side from time to time. We talked about the difference between medication-induced hallucinations, and reality-based visitations from loved ones who had already passed on.

As her body continued to fail, Valerie remained clear-thinking and began talking more about her funeral, reminding me that after the service, there would be lots of "eats." I asked if she would like me to sing at her funeral and she said yes. Together we previewed a variety of songs, and she chose "In the Garden." I told her that singing would be my final gift to her. She thought for a moment and then broke into a broad grin as she said I was to eat as much food as I wanted at her funeral for that would be *her* final gift to *me*.

One of our most fun visits together occurred in December. Her latest concern was whether or not her funeral outfit would still look good on her. She asked me to help her try it on, which, due to her debilitated state, was totally out of the question. I retrieved the outfit from the closet and saw that the two-piece skirt suit was a size 8 and had never been worn. It had a short-sleeved classy sweater to match; however, one of her family members had replaced it with a gray silk blouse they thought might be fancier. We decided that I should model each piece and give her a fashion show! So, while Elton was at the grocery store, the two of us laughed and carried on like teenagers at a pajama party.

The gray blouse was hideously large and bulked up by big shoulder pads, not to mention the ugly neckline. Valerie gave it a thumbs down. The sweater was so elegant that we both knew immediately that it was a keeper. We went through 18 scarves in her top dresser drawer until we found one that coordinated all the colors. She told me to put the outfit on a hanger with a dry cleaning bag over it for protection. I was to mark on a piece of masking tape that this was the outfit Valerie wanted to be buried in, with no substitutions! She then had me hide the ugly gray blouse in the back of the coat closet where she hoped no one would find it until after she was "long gone."

She directed me to get out an ecru colored afghan-like shawl from the hope chest. She asked to be interred with the shawl over her shoulders because she was "always cold." However, she said emphatically, "Do not put it on me when I am laid out because I'd look stupid, and I intend to be the best-dressed woman at my own funeral!" She later added that she'd like to have leg-warmers on before she was buried and, at the end, I honored this request.

Midway through December, Valerie again informed me that she had no intention of dying over the holidays and ruining them "like her father did." Although I didn't comment, I couldn't help but wonder how her frail body could possibly live much longer. But, with her iron will, Valerie seemed to rally somewhat, despite a recently placed catheter.

She actually got dressed and had family members help her walk to the living room recliner one evening when a group of hospice volunteers came Christmas caroling. According to Valerie, if death wanted her, it would have to wait.

My next few visits found Valerie in the living room recliner, glad to be out of bed, and eager to write letters to close family members. She was too weak to write them herself, so she would dictate the contents and I would write the notes. She'd start by thanking them for helping her in some way, but not know what else to say. I'd try prompting her to remember a specific incident that might have pertained to her relationship with that particular person. She'd slay me with her witty remarks, and the two of us would laugh until our sides hurt. She'd come up with things we couldn't possibly write down, such as remembering how her brother used to hide behind a cherry tree to soil his pants! Or, that a sister would bring her a pie and then take half of it back home with her! Needless to say, those letters took awhile to complete, but we did have fun, and it got her talking about her youth again. I wrote them out in longhand, and then held her arm steady while she signed them.

After the Christmas holidays, Valerie again became weak and bedridden. She fussed about all she still needed to do, like packing up items, or sorting through recipes but it was obvious that those chores weren't possible. We talked about how she needed to let go of earthly matters and focus on what she needed to do to make the transition. After the New Year, a nasty bout of diarrhea seemed to weaken her spirit as well as her body. Body hygiene had always been very important to her and we both realized the end was drawing near.

On my next Tuesday visit, I had a sore throat and therefore sat far enough away from Valerie not to spread my germs. By Wednesday, I had come down with a full-blown cold and realized I couldn't go to see Valerie the next day. We don't visit patients when we are sick as it can compromise their weakened immune systems. Between blowing my nose, sneezing and coughing, I wrestled with my emotions about not getting to see her for our regularly scheduled Thursday visit. I knew I needed to call Elton and cancel the next day's visit, but I kept putting it off until it became too late that night to call. The next morning I was up early but knew I couldn't call Elton until after 9 a.m. as they were late risers. What happened next is truly unexplainable.

As I sat at my kitchen table, I began feeling very sleepy. I thought if I took a 10-minute nap while I was waiting to call, I might feel better. I went to the bedroom and laid down on top of my bedspread, glancing at the digital clock on the dresser before closing my eyes. It said 8:00 a.m. I instantly fell asleep and found myself in a garden setting. I was standing in a small courtyard that held two curved cement benches. There was an arched rose trellis that led into the main garden area. I was aware of the presence of three angels, two female and one male, although I couldn't see their faces, only white hazy forms. One took my clothes, folded and laid them on one of the benches. I was given a long white gown to put on that was high-waisted and short-sleeved. One of the angels extended her arm to me, palm side down, and somehow I knew I was to place my hand over hers so I could be led somewhere. When I asked where we were going, she mentally conveyed, "to the Hall of Healing." I looked up to see a magnificent white building atop a small hill. The building appeared to glow with bright white energy. That was the last thing I remembered before waking up and seeing the digital clock which now said 8:35 a.m. I sat up on the bed and realized instantly that my cold was gone. No mucous, no swollen glands, no sore throat, no coughing, no sneezing —nothing! I dropped to my knees in shock and thanked God for this miracle.

At 1:15 p.m., I arrived at Valerie's apartment for our Thursday scheduled time together. She and I had a wonderful visit which turned out to be our last, as she passed away the following Monday after slipping into a coma. Valerie had been very fearful of dying while trying to catch her breath, so I was glad to hear from the hospice nurse that she had died gently.

Both my husband and I attended Valerie's viewing. I was pleased to see that her hair and makeup was as beautiful as she had hoped, and that her funeral outfit looked great. Oddly enough, though, there was a pungent perfume smell at the viewing that seemed to follow us. I thought perhaps it had been the overwhelmingly fragrant flowers at the viewing or someone wearing too much cologne. However, the smell lingered in our car on the drive home, although my husband's usually sensitive nose didn't smell the odor. I suspected the odor had gotten into my clothes, and I was somewhat irritated by this annoyance. The smell was still with me as I got into bed, which is when I had an "aha" moment that maybe the smell was a "sign." To rule out this possibility, I said aloud, "If that's you Val, thank you for letting me know you still exist." The smell disappeared instantly.

At Valerie's funeral the next day, I sang "In the Garden," which now had an even deeper meaning for me since the spiritual dream experience of the prior week. During the service, I spoke of some of my special memories of Valerie and shared some of our mutual experiences, including the laughs we shared. After the service, I passed along the letters she had written to each of her family members.

The hospice nurse, social worker, and I attended the luncheon in the church's main hall that Valerie had prearranged. I made sure to get plenty of "eats" as she had wanted me to do. A funny incident occurred while we were eating. Three little old ladies came shuffling over to our table, arms linked and clutching their handbags. They asked for my phone number, saying that when they were dying, they wanted to have fun with a hospice volunteer like Valerie did!

Elton called me the following week to let me know that he and some of Valerie's siblings had gone to New York State where a second funeral service had been held for her. Because it had been a mild winter, the grave site could be dug, and Valerie had been given the proper burial she had wanted.

Case #7

UNOFFICIAL VOLUNTEER

Bertha was the wife of my second Hospice client, Anthony. I noticed her sitting in the foyer of the assisted living facility where I conducted Monday sing-alongs. She had been losing weight steadily since Anthony died of prostate cancer six months prior. They had been married for over sixty years, and she told me she felt lost without him. Her sons had moved Bertha to the first floor of this same assisted living facility that the couple shared when he was living, hoping the familiarity would afford her friendships and comfort.

I decided to see Bertha on an unofficial basis. She remembered me vaguely but, due to her advancing dementia, we talked only about current happenings. Bertha had been a piano teacher all her life, which was something we had in common. I began visiting her privately on Mondays for an hour, and then she would accompany me to the sing-alongs. Although she couldn't remember my name on each visit, she would recognize my face and our common love of music.

One Monday at the conclusion of a sing-along, I assisted Bertha to the piano bench and asked her to play something. For a moment, she couldn't remember what to do. Then, suddenly, her hands began to bounce along the black keys while she sang, "I like coffee, I like tea, I like the boys and the boys like me!" I joined her on the bench for a duet, playing the treble clef high notes while she played the low notes. We had a good laugh while staff members clapped encouragingly.

Unfortunately, Bertha had a tumor growing on the side of her face at an alarming rate. The tumor was cancerous, and radiation treatments were begun in an effort to shrink it. The treatments took a toll on her body and eventually she was too weak to attend the sing-alongs. We stayed in her room during my visits. She would lie back in her recliner, very tired and frail. One afternoon, Bertha patted my hand and closed her eyes, drifting into a semi-sleep while I sat on the floor next to her chair. I sang hymn after hymn as she held my hand. When I stopped singing, she opened her eyes and said faintly, "Am I in heaven?" I laughed and said, "No, Bertha. Trust me—when you get to heaven, the music will be much prettier!" We both laughed.

Shortly after this incident, radiation treatments were discontinued and Bertha was admitted to Hospice care. I was officially assigned as her volunteer. Sadly, I only got to visit her once in this capacity. It was a Friday at noontime. She was semi-comatose with one son sitting next to her bed holding her hand. He had come on his lunch hour to be with her. He and I talked for a few minutes about his mother and then he went back to work. Bertha was not physically aware of my presence.

Her body was very restless in the bed, and I suspected she was actively dying. I talked quietly to her, letting her know how much I had enjoyed knowing her. I sang our sing-along repertoire softly a cappella, telling her how much she'd be missed. I then quietly played one of our favorite Chopin tapes on my cassette player. When the tape finished, I kissed her and left. She passed away later that evening.

Case #8

TIMELESSNESS

I was still missing Bertha when I was assigned my next patient, Harold. The "get to know you" visitation occurred on a Friday. Harold was a widower, living in his own home, in the same town in which I lived. As hospice requires each patient to have a caretaker, Harold's son, Ned, was temporarily living with him.

Harold was lying on the living room couch with a bedside commode next to him when I arrived. We had a nice conversation about his former government job. I admired the beautiful framed medallion necklace that hung on the wall, an honor given him by a fraternal organization to which he belonged. He was proud to tell me about this necklace, although he did so in a very weary-sounding voice.

I was supposed to return on Monday to sit

with Harold for four hours while Ned ran errands, but Ned called to cancel my visit. He said his father had had a bad weekend. By Ned's report, Harold had been too weak to get up by himself to use the commode and, while assisting him, both men had fallen. Luckily, neither was badly injured, although Ned had to summon paramedic assistance to get Harold back into bed.

On Tuesday, I stayed with Harold for three hours while Ned went to work. A catheterized Harold now lay in a hospital bed, which had been set up in the living room. He occasionally responded to my questions with one-word answers, but mostly he drifted into and out of sleep. I sat next to his bed, singing songs from the 1930's and 1940's, and then spoke softly to him about his worn out body. I explained that loved ones would be waiting on the Other Side to greet him and that his earthly family here had great memories of him to cherish. The hours seemed to evaporate as I experienced an odd sensation of timelessness while by his bedside.

The following day, Ned called to say that Harold had passed away.

I wondered if the timelessness experienced the previous day had come back for him.

Case #9

SONGBIRD

This was the second time I'd been asked by hospice to supplement a family's regular volunteer. Esther, a scleroderma patient, lived with her son, daughter-in-law, and 12-year-old granddaughter, Leah, in a town nearby. The primary volunteer visited on Thursdays, but the family had asked for more assistance as the son's wife, Nicole, suffered from depression and the stress of caring for her mother-in-law full-time.

Nicole and Leah were very welcoming on my first visit. We stood in the kitchen and talked about their situation. Prior to entering hospice, Esther had lived in their basement, but recently, the family had moved her into Leah's first-floor bedroom, where she could watch a birdfeeder stationed outside the window. Leah was temporarily sleeping on the floor of her parent's bedroom, while their newly acquired puppy slept in the basement. The house was very small. The family had no television. Nicole said they were strongly committed Christians who listened to religious audiotapes and watched the birds in their spare time.

Nicole said her husband was a hard worker who put in long hours, so the caregiving duties fell on her shoulders. She admitted she was struggling under the burden. They had installed an intercom in order to hear and converse with Esther when the family was in another room.

We mutually agreed that I would visit on Mondays from 12:30 until 3 p.m., and on Fridays from 2 to 4, so Nicole could run errands while Leah was in school.

On my initial visit, Nicole and Leah (both petite) commented on my 5-foot 10-inch height. When we entered Esther's bedroom, she said something about my size also. She then asked me to sit in a rocking chair at the foot of her bed. Nicole and Leah left to go shopping, so I was on my own. The bedroom was exceptionally tiny and crowded; however, it was painted a bright yellow and had two windows which provided a cheerful atmosphere. Esther was clear-headed and looked in fairly good physical shape. She had a bedside commode for she was too weak to walk to the bathroom by herself. She said either Nicole or a hospice home health care aide would bathe her in bed. Before accepting this case, I had been advised by my supervisor that the patient also suffered emotionally from OCD (obsessive compulsive disorder) and had a "germ" phobia. There would be no hugging or touching on this case, and I would have to be sensitive to the patient's fears.

Although Nicole had mentioned that Esther might want me to read religious literature to her because she was weak and tired, instead, to my delight, Esther talked non-stop for two hours. She told me about her early life and the course of her disease, scleroderma, which had been present for over thirty years. She asked me some personal questions about myself, and I was straightforward in my replies. She asked to be called "Essie" and we talked about the origin of her germ phobia. It seems a friend had made a remark about people spitting on sidewalks and germs being brought into homes on people's feet, and Essie's phobia had blossomed from there. I made sure to wash my hands twice with antibacterial hand cleaner to reassure her while I sat and listened. She asked about the cleaner and I explained that it could be used without water. She was very interested in it and I later brought some for her personal use.

On my second visit, Nicole mentioned that Essie had asked when "Six-Foot-Linda" was coming back. We laughed, and I made it a point to identify myself that way whenever I phoned. The family said Essie didn't usually warm up to strangers, so they were pleased that she seemed to like me. They told me that earlier in the week, Essie had fallen over the toiletry table, which had been next to the commode. She had suffered minor bruising and a scraped heel. We then proceeded to Essie's bedroom and were in there when the hospice nurse arrived.

Although the nurse put on gloves, Essie wouldn't let her pull back the covers; instead, she did it herself. Essie also removed her own sock, as she really didn't want the nurse to touch her. Essie got very nervous and sharp-tongued with the nurse who was in close proximity. The nurse said Essie's foot was a little spongy and needed to be elevated with the heel hung over a pillow, which Essie insisted on doing herself. Just before leaving, the nurse accidentally stepped on a slipper that was next to the bed, and Essie yelled at her for "contaminating it." After the nurse left, I distracted Essie by talking about how hospice could provide a sturdier commode to keep her safer and, although hesitant, she agreed it might be a good idea. I called the office to arrange delivery when I got home.

The new commode was there on my third visit, and Essie appeared pleased with its added height. A genuine feeling of camaraderie seemed to emerge between us that day. Essie asked about some of my other hospice experiences. When she found out I could sing, she mentioned that there were several hymns in her religious songbook that she loved, and she regretted not being able to get out to the Kingdom Hall to hear them anymore. I looked at her hymn book and suggested that I bring my keyboard on the next visit so I could play the melodies. She agreed.

I must have been quite a sight upon entering Essie's little bedroom on my next visit, struggling with a full-sized keyboard, which I assured her had been sanitized before I entered. I sat in the rocker, balanced the keyboard on my knees, held her hymnal in my left hand, and played melodies with my right. Essie had dog-eared the pages of her favorite hymns, so I was able to go from one to another smoothly. Once I became familiar with the melodies, I suggested that we sing them together, which we did. The three-hour visit flew by.

News about the keyboard and hymn singing must have spread quickly in the household because when Leah got home from school on a subsequent visit, she asked me to stay a little longer so she could join in the singing. Even Nicole, upon arriving home from running errands, sang with us. We had a grand time, and Essie seemed alert and well. Before leaving, I explained that I wouldn't be visiting the following week as I would be on a family vacation.

When I returned from vacation, a message on my answering machine from Nicole said that Essie was actively dying. I returned the call and learned that Essie's eyes were closed and her respirations shallow, but she wouldn't let go and the family worried that it might be because I hadn't said goodbye. Her regular volunteer had already stopped by to do so. I explained to Nicole that my sister, a registered nurse, was staying with me for a few days, and I asked if we could both visit the next day. Nicole agreed and asked me to bring my keyboard along.

My sister and I arrived at 10 a.m. the following day. I met Essie's son for the first time. He and his wife had been sitting vigil with her all night. They told us they would remain in the kitchen so that I could say my goodbyes privately. My sister and I entered the bedroom, and my sister sat quietly in a chair off to the side. Although Essie's eyes were shut and she appeared to be asleep, I stood next to the bed and told her I was there. I also told her how much I had enjoyed getting to know her and how we all loved her. I told her we wanted her to let go and die peacefully. I jokingly said I'd play and sing her favorite hymns as a send off. I spent a half hour playing the keyboard and singing. My sister told me that she saw Essie's lips moving to one of the tunes, although her eyes had remained closed. After our visit, my sister and I went to the kitchen to talk to the family for a few minutes. Nicole shared that the previous week, Essie had stopped calling me "Six-Foot-Linda" and instead had referred to me as her "Songbird." I was very touched.

The following day, the family called to say Essie had passed away peacefully around 5 o'clock that morning.

Case #10

TRUST MY INSTINCTS

My next patient, like Essie, was an elderly widowed woman. Her name was Iris. She had suffered a massive stroke and had recently been discharged from a city hospital to a nursing home in the town in which her son lived. She had another child, a daughter, who lived out West.

An assigned hospice volunteer visited evenings but the family had requested an additional volunteer to visit during the day.

Iris was lying on her right side facing the window of her semiprivate room when I arrived for my first visit. Her roommate's bed was empty. Iris's left side was paralyzed, and she kept extending her right hand through the bars of the bed railing as if asking to have it held.

Despite her advanced age, Iris's face was relatively unlined and her long, lovely gray hair fanned out on the pillow. A loud oxygen machine droned in the background with yards of tubing lying across the bed culminating at the nasal cannula. Iris couldn't speak but had beautiful expressive pale blue eyes. I held her right hand and explained that I was one of her hospice volunteers —her daytime "singing volunteer." I had brought written song sheets with me as I never was good at memorizing words. I sang softly into her right ear until she fell asleep.

An hour later, the patient's daughter, Evelyn, entered the room unexpectedly. We were both surprised to find one another there. I had been told that the daughter, who had flown into town when notified of her mother's stroke, had returned to Nebraska. I explained who I was, and Evelyn told me that every time she got to the airport, she "wouldn't feel right" and would return to her mother's bedside. To me, Evelyn seemed very agitated and sleep deprived. I asked if things were progressing all right for her, and she replied "not really." She said the transition of her mother into hospice care had been "rocky" and she wasn't pleased. This was my first experience in having someone complain about hospice. Just then, an aide came into the room to reposition Iris, so I suggested to Evelyn that we go elsewhere to talk. There was an empty hospital bed in the hallway outside the room, so Evelyn and I sat there conversing for 40 minutes. The frustrations poured out of her. It seemed she didn't like the hospice nurse assigned to the case and, in probing further, it really sounded like a miscommunication. According to Evelyn, when the hospice nurse first visited, Iris had messed herself. The nurse had asked Evelyn to assist by holding Iris's legs while she cleaned her up, and Evelyn had been horrified at participating in such a task. Furthermore, she felt the nurse had rushed the rest of the visit. Evelyn had called her brother, who lived nearby, to complain, and he had asked her not to cause trouble for the family. As power-of-attorney, he told her he would be the one having to deal with everything after she left. Evelyn was still angry at hospice and her brother.

While she talked, I was reminded of what we learned in hospice training about "unfinished business" and how it could prevent patients from making their final transitions. I wondered if it could be family discord holding Iris back. After Evelyn finished her recitation of grievances, I explained the overall purpose of hospice and assured her that we all wanted the same thing—a peaceful transition for her mother. I urged her to call and share her concerns with the hospice nurse so that her issues could be resolved to everyone's satisfaction. She seemed hesitant to do so and said that maybe she had just needed to get her resentments out in the open. I wrote down my name and phone number and said she could call me any time she wanted to talk. We hugged and she seemed calm by the time I left.

I returned to Iris's room the following afternoon. I stayed with her for over two hours, singing most of the time. When I first arrived, she grabbed at my hand, but when I started singing, she relaxed. I got the feeling she knew why I was there and was beginning to feel comfortable with me. Her daughter, Evelyn, never visited again while I was there. I wondered if she had finally flown back home.

Two days later when I entered the room, Iris seemed very agitated. Not only did she grab my hand, she kept digging her nails into my palm. Although unable to talk, her actions were saying something was wrong. I tried singing to calm her but it had no effect. I walked down to the nurses' station to share my concerns. The nurse was on break but two aides came back to the room with me. As they were re-positioning her catheter bag, they noticed the nasal cannula tubing had become crimped, cutting off her oxygen supply.

The next hour was spent with staff replacing the oxygen canister and tubing so that air could flow freely again. I had hoped that Iris would settle down and relax after the machine was fixed, but she continued to rake my palm with her nails. A licensed practical nurse came in to administer Morphine and Ativan under her tongue, which Iris instantly opened her mouth to accept. It took 40 more minutes before she drifted off to sleep. Intuitively, I felt as if she had begun the active dying process. While she slept, I checked her fingernail and toenail beds for any bluing, but they looked pink and normal. She had no mottling on her arms or legs to suggest limited circulation. I still felt uncomfortable with the situation, so when I got home, I phoned the hospice nurse to relay my concerns.

Two days later, I got a call from hospice advising me that Iris had died peacefully the preceding evening. So, despite not having the physical symptoms normally present when active dying has begun, Iris died anyway! Note to self: trust my instincts.

Case #11

GARDEN CONNECTION

My eleventh case, Connie, had been referred through a mutual friend; they had been in a cancer support group together. When Connie's ovarian/ breast cancer returned with a vengeance, and the doctors had no further treatment options to offer, she entered hospice. That's when our mutual friend recommended that she request me as her volunteer.

On my initial visit in March, Connie greeted me at the front door of her beautiful country home looking cheerful and well. She was tall and tanned, with short, thick grey hair. Connie said she wasn't even sure she needed hospice care yet, but quality of life issues mattered to her and, if hospice could help, "so be it." I learned that she was three years older than I and we shared a common interest in golf and reading.

We had a leisurely chat while seated in the library section of her home. Connie said she had undergone yearly PAP smears and mammograms; therefore, two years ago, it came as a shock when a routine mammogram showed a Stage II cancer. At the pre-op physical preceding her scheduled mastectomy, Connie mentioned to the doctor that she was having bouts of diarrhea alternating with constipation. He ordered an ultrasound of her abdomen, which revealed a cancerous ovarian tumor wrapped around her bowel. The mastectomy was cancelled and surgery was performed to remove the ovarian tumor.

When Connie recovered from that surgery, she had a breast lumpectomy followed by chemotherapy. After the treatments ended, Connie felt well enough to resume playing golf in her ladies league. This lasted for four months before she had to stop due to weakness. At that time, a CT scan revealed that the cancer had metastasized and further chemotherapy ensued. Connie developed allergies to those treatments and grew tired of the numerous side effects. She opted to discontinue treatment and enter hospice.

Connie said her husband Hank, who was retired, supported her decision. She said he was a kind, loving man who had his own problems, as his mother suffered from cancer also. Connie said she was disappointed in her hospital cancer support group because most of the members saw her entry into hospice as "giving up." They felt she should have researched alternative therapies on the Internet. This led to our discussion about how differently people react to terminal illnesses. After our chat, we mutually agreed that I'd return the following week.

On my second visit, Connie and I sat at her kitchen table. Her nephew had visited over the weekend, and she said that although she loved him, company seemed to wear her out. The nephew's brother had since called and asked if he and his family could come visit, and Connie felt obligated to say yes. We explored her feelings, and I encouraged her to put her own needs first. She was uncomfortable with the concept and felt that she should entertain, regardless of how it made her feel. It gave us a chance to talk about "shoulds." I shared some comments a Hospice speaker had made about not letting others "should" all over us. We both laughed. We then talked about how others are often uncomfortable with the issue of dying; how they don't know what to say, what to do, or how to act, and how we all stumble through this final journey.

Ten days elapsed before my next visit due to scheduling conflicts for both of us. Connie seemed a bit weaker and paler. More relatives had visited. We shared pleasantries, and then she surprised me by saying that she didn't want anyone around her once she became bedridden.

Connie went on to say that this included her husband, family, friends, and any hospice personnel. She said she didn't want further discussion about it, so we talked lightly about other things before I left.

Two weeks passed before I saw Connie again. I wanted to see her twice weekly, but she kept canceling our visits. The lack of continuity wasn't helping us bond, although things improved one day when we sat on her screened-in porch and played cards. I taught her a game called "Golf," a quick and easy card game that has nine hands, called "holes." Being an avid golfer, she thought that playing "nine holes of golf" with the cards was cute and fun. It was a lovely May afternoon, and we watched the birds at the feeder in-between deals. Our conversation was light, but she did mention going on pain medication. The cancer had metastasized to her lymphatic system now, and small tumors had formed along her rib cage. She was having bowel problems also, which irked her more than anything.

I visited the following week, but due to cold weather, we stayed in her kitchen. I told Connie about our 33 year-old, single head-strong daughter, who had gotten engaged over the weekend. We laughed about God having someone for everyone. Connie had married for the first time in her mid-thirties also. Conversation flowed from one topic to another and we both shared stories of interesting unusual family members. She talked about a male cousin who had been abusive to his wife all his life until he had gotten a terminal illness. Connie said that through him, she had learned a valuable lesson, which was to "never kick your caregiver." We both laughed so hard that we doubled over and kept repeating the phrase, "Never kick your caregiver." We then shared stores about women who had made passes at our husbands. Connie said she hoped her husband would remarry when she was gone so he'd have companionship. She also said she hoped that her husband could "tell her to go" when the time came. She worried about this because two weeks earlier, her husband couldn't say those words to his dying mother despite hospice literature he had read which had urged him to do so.

I only visited Connie once in the next month due to family commitments for both of us. When next I saw her, she was lying on her bed due to a backache. I pulled up a chair and proceeded to amuse her with tales of family shenanigans that had occurred on my recent trip to Florida. We both laughed a lot. We agreed to meet again in two weeks, but Connie cancelled that visit. She said she was "going downhill physically" and recently had gotten a hospital bed and commode. She said that all these changes were exhausting, and she didn't want company. I really wanted to help her and felt frustrated to be turned away.

The next day I prayed for guidance and got an inspiration. The pansies in the little sidewalk garden by Connie's mailbox had died from the hot weather. As Connie and I regularly communicated by e-mail, I sent her a message that I'd like to fix up her sidewalk garden, as it was something I could do without bothering her, which would make us both feel better. I said if I didn't hear from her by e-mail or phone saying not to come, I would stop by in two days to garden. Early in the morning two days later, I knelt by Connie's mailbox and was engrossed in planting dianthus and mums when she opened the front door and asked what I was doing there. It was an awkward moment. Then, she told me to come sit next to her on the porch bench. As I explained the situation, she said she hadn't checked her e-mail in two days due to exhaustion.

Instead of being angry with me, she was touched by my offering. Under her watchful eye, I spent the next two hours completing the job. The flowers seemed to cheer her and the following week, we e-mailed back and forth about our mutual interest in gardening.

On our next visit, we seemed to have found a

new comfort level with one another. Connie reclined on the living room couch while I sat in an
armchair. She hesitated a moment and then told
me she had seen both her parents standing in the
living room the previous day. As both her parents
had died when she was 12, Connie questioned
whether or not the vision had been real or imag-
ined. It gave us an opportunity to talk about life after death and the possibility that loved ones could
greet us when we crossed over. She said two
of her aunts had died of ovarian cancer and that
sometimes when she got discouraged with pain
or nausea, she felt them sitting nearby encouraging her. We talked about the importance of humor
in keeping spirits up. We discovered that both of
us admired comedian Lily Tomlin. I started doing an impersonation of Tomlin's "Ernestine," and
Connie laughed so hard she asked me to stop my
performance so she could catch her breath. I left
when the hospice home health aide showed up for
Connie's bath, but not before we mutually agreed
on regular Tuesday morning visits at 10 a.m..

On our next visit, we talked in her bedroom.
I lounged on the queen-sized bed across from her
hospital bed. Connie mentioned that whenever
she went out to eat with her husband, the next day
she'd be exhausted. She noticed her energy level
had diminished greatly. Then we talked about the
book I had lent her the previous week called *Mes-*

sages from Heaven. It was about a deceased man who talks to his wife from the Other Side. He tells her what life is like in heaven and philosophizes about it. Connie found the book comforting and mentally stimulating. She subsequently called the publisher and ordered a copy for herself so she could highlight passages. On this visit, Connie seemed more tired than usual and her complexion looked sallow. We agreed that I would continue to garden on Fridays, and make in-person visits to her on Tuesdays.

The following Friday, I parked behind the house and immersed myself in pruning the two huge butterfly bushes near the kitchen, trimming off the expired blooms so new ones could develop. An hour after beginning this project, Connie came out onto the adjacent screened-in porch. She called out to me that she wanted to discuss the "heaven book" further, so I pruned while she talked.

The next Tuesday, Connie seemed washed out. She reminisced more than usual. She said Hank felt she had been confused and forgetful recently, and he wondered if it could be due to her medications. She disagreed, saying it was because she "didn't sweat the small stuff anymore." We talked about how one must let go of earthly matters in order to make preparations for arriving on the Other Side. Our conversation was informal and relaxed. I sensed a new calm in her.

In August, Connie's face looked smaller as she had lost weight. The hospice nurse had prescribed a diuretic to get rid of excess tumor fluid. Connie was happy that she felt lighter but complained of two new pains; one was a chest pain in the heart region, and the other was a knee pain. Of the two, the knee pain bothered her the most. She said it felt like bone on bone with something swirling around inside. At my urging, she phoned the hospice nurse and left a message about the new pains. Then, she reclined on her hospital bed as I sat across from her. She requested information about water fountains as she wanted to donate one to the new inpatient hospice facility that was being built in our town. She wanted the fountain to be small so it could stay indoors. She hoped hospice clients would sit beside it and feel soothed. We also talked about my oldest daughter's upcoming October wedding, and Connie said she wanted to still be alive in order to hear how everything turned out. She mentioned that four of her golfing buddies had stopped by the previous Friday. Her husband had made lunch for all of them. Connie was glad the focus had been on sharing laughter and golf experiences rather than talking about her cancer.

Another week went by, and Connie said she had lost 30 pounds on the diuretic, making her feel less bulky. She seemed somewhat confused, not being able to stay on one topic without a cross-over of words. I showed her the dress I planned to wear to my daughter's wedding, and she loved it. She asked that I take lots of pictures. She then switched subjects and said she wanted to talk about the drawing I had shown her the previous week. The drawing had been one I made in a hospice class where the assignment had been to draw what we thought our entry into death would look like. Connie said she wanted to draw how she thought her own moment of death would be. I got out some paper and a pencil but her hand was too shaky to manage the task.

Despite my protests that I could only draw stick figures, she insisted I draw the scene for her. She described herself sitting on a chair in a room while being greeted by her two deceased aunts. She told me to put a light source in the left hand corner (I drew a sun) and in the right-hand corner, she wanted her parents to be standing. We discussed the picture afterwards. She said she was angry with her parents so she wanted them in the corner, with them not knowing whether to enter the room or not. She said she had been 12 years old when her mother had died from alcoholism.

Her father died shortly thereafter from the same disease. After their deaths, Connie had gone to live with her father's sister (one of the aunts in the picture). This aunt eventually died from ovarian cancer. Connie got very emotional and shared many feelings of anger, resentment, and sadness towards her parents.

In September, Connie greeted me with the question, "Am I a fraud?" She was lounging on her hospital bed while I sat in a chair next to her. She expressed some confusion about the dying process. She said she had expected to be dead by now. She quizzed me with questions I couldn't answer, such as: "Am I really sick? Why haven't the tumors gotten the best of me yet?" I told her that often patients got better or remained stable with good pain control and medical management when they entered hospice; it wasn't unusual. I went on to say that perhaps by not having additional chemotherapy, her body's immune system wasn't as compromised. She mentioned bouts of constipation that continued to plague her, although she had gotten relief from stool softeners and enemas over the weekend. I encouraged her to discuss these issues with her hospice nurse who could properly answer her questions.

The following Tuesday, Connie was weaker, but could still walk. Hank had hired a private duty nurse's aide, Latisha, to bathe her daily and help around the house. Connie liked Latisha very much. I had brought Connie a copy of a book I was reading—a lovely sentimental novel. She promised to read a chapter to see if it "grabbed" her but did point out that she was behind in her reading as people kept bringing more books.

On my next visit, Connie told me her brother had stopped in for an overnight stay as he had been on a business trip in the area. She had been thrilled to see him. They had discussed their early family life together. When she told me about the visit, she positively glowed. She had read the first chapter of the novel I had given her but said she kept getting "fuzzy" which made concentration hard.

Four days later, there was a new medical development. Connie said a band of tumors in her lower abdomen seemed to shake, causing an odd sensation, like Jell-O jiggling. It didn't hurt her, but the pulsating movement made the cancer seem alive, which scared her.

Mid-September marked Connie's 23rd wedding anniversary. I brought a cut flower arrangement from a local market with me. The bouquet featured two large sunflowers, which seemed to brighten up the living room. Connie said she and her husband had postponed their dinner celebration, as she had been too tired to leave the house. It seems she had gone to lunch with Latisha the previous day, and the outing had exhausted her.

On my next visit, Connie's "fuzziness" had cleared up, and she was happy to be thinking and speaking clearly again. The problem had been with taking medication dosages improperly. To correct the problem, the hospice nurse had drawn up syringes with the appropriate dosages to be administered directly into Connie's mouth at scheduled times. This new oral dosing routine worked out well, and Connie's confusion resolved.

In late September, Connie invited me to her home for a birthday luncheon hosted by her husband. The hospice nurse and social worker were there also, having brought Connie a vase of yellow roses. Latisha had set the table with pretty plates and table linens, and Hank had ordered Chinese food. I brought an ice cream cake. I knew Connie would enjoy it because on a previous visit, she had shown me her large upright freezer. Inside the freezer were twenty gallons of ice cream in assorted flavors. Connie loved ice cream and had decided when she was diagnosed as 'terminal' that she would eat ice cream whenever she felt like it. This sounded like a great plan to me! As for Connie's birthday party, her favorite cousin, Celia, who lived on the Eastern Shore, arrived a little late, but with her usual flare. Celia reminded us all of the character "Auntie Mame." Celia was dressed in a long bright orange dress, with matching hat and socks, a wardrobe befitting her work as an artist. She entertained us with stories of their exciting youth together, since she and Connie had been raised as sisters when Connie's parents died. The six of us sat around the kitchen table getting to know one another better with Connie officiating, very content to be among the people with whom she felt the most relaxed. We had all heard of one another but it was nice to put faces with names.

The beginning of October, Connie still used a walker but spent more time in bed. She had read a hospice publication called "Crossing the Creek," which explained in detailed stages the physical transition process for dying. Again, Connie was full of questions. She wanted to know why her progress towards death seemed to be at a standstill. She asked if her cancer "had taken a holiday?" She said she felt pressure in her swollen abdomen but her appetite was still good, so "what was the deal?" I quipped, "Remember when Jesus said, 'I go to prepare a place for you?' Well, maybe your room isn't ready yet!" We both laughed. After that comment, Connie napped for two hours while I went outside to tidy up the butterfly bushes on the side of the house.

I didn't see Connie again for two weeks as I had gone to California for our daughter's wedding. On a subsequent visit, Connie seemed disappointed that I hadn't brought any photos with me. I sensed she had begun a downhill slide physically. She was somewhat agitated, and her pain level had increased. I was glad the hospice nurse arrived while I was still there. The nurse said the tumors were actively growing, and Connie's medications needed to be increased. Connie surprised us both by saying she was worried about being able to climb the stairs into heaven since her physical body had gotten so heavy with tumors and fluid recently. After the nurse and aide left the room, Connie and I talked about how light her soul body would be after she died, and how the soul body would be the one to carry her to heaven.

The moment I entered her room on our mid-October visit, Connie reached for the wedding photos I had brought. She studied each picture like it was a treasure; however, after every two photos, she would nod off to sleep. Her legs and feet looked very swollen to me. Cousin Celia and aide Latisha arrived halfway through my visit. Connie awoke and shared some vivid dreams she'd been having, including one about colorful chickens and seeing a bright light. No mention was made of deceased relatives though, which was really what she wanted to experience.

How quickly things changed in a week! The following Tuesday, Connie was more out of it than with it. She said hi and recognized me when I arrived, but quickly drifted off to sleep. Her nail beds looked clear, but her husband said her back was mottled. On the lighter side, when I bent over the bed to ask Connie if she wanted me to sing to her,

she opened her eyes and gave me a loud, "NO!"
Instead, I read aloud passages she had highlighted
from her favorite book (the one about heaven).

Another week passed before I saw Connie
again. This time I brought a cassette tape by Bel-
leruth Naparstek called "Peaceful Dying." The
hospice nurse had been flushing Connie's port
when I arrived, so I stayed in the living room with
Latisha, who gave me an update on Connie's decline. When the nurse left, the hospice chaplain
arrived for a private visit. When the chaplain left,
Latisha and I finally were able to visit with Connie,
who didn't open her eyes or respond when we said
her name. We suspected she might be in the active dying process, so Latisha and I sat on opposite
sides of the hospital bed, with each of us holding
one of Connie's hands. We let the meditation cassette tape play quietly in the background. We each
told her we loved her. We could see a fluttering
underneath her eyelids, and a rise and fall of her
chest when we talked. We hoped she would die
gently while listening to the tape surrounded by
our love; however, she remained peacefully alive.

Three days later as I was getting ready to visit
Connie, I received a call from the hospice nurse
saying that Connie had passed away early that
morning after a brief bout of respiratory distress.
I spent the rest of the day thinking about Connie
and typing up my hospice notes. I tried to sit qui-

etly in my rocking chair while checking for grammatical errors, but the clock over our fireplace mantel ticked so loudly that it kept interrupting my concentration. At the time, I thought it odd that I had never noticed how loud that clock could get. I gave up and went to bed.

The following day when I went down to our family room to resume the edit, I immediately noticed that I couldn't hear the clock ticking. I sat very still and strained my ears, but the clock was not audible. Had the loud ticking been Connie's way of letting me know she was okay?

The following Tuesday, I made my regular visit to Connie's home but this time, it was for a bereavement visit to her husband. Before I had a chance to share my news about the clock's loud ticking, Hank told me about an odd incident that had occurred the day Connie died. At 10 a.m., the morning of her passing, all the phones in the house stopped working. The phone repair crew that came to investigate the problem could find no explanation. The phones began working again after they left. Hank wondered if it was Connie's way of saying goodbye to him.

On Sunday at 3 p.m., a memorial service for Connie was held at the Episcopal Church in town. She had designed the service herself. The day was heavily overcast with intermittent showers. The church was filled to capacity with friends and family. The service began with a taped Gospel song by Anne Murray. As soon as the song began, a sunbeam streamed through an upper stained glass window, despite the dark black sky. An audible gasp rippled through the church.

After the mass, all in attendance were treated to a catered dinner at a local restaurant. About twelve to fifteen tables of ten had been set up and filled rapidly. At our table, my husband and I were joined by two of Connie's cancer support group friends, her brother, and her cousin, Celia. Everyone was eager to share stories about Connie. The group of us alternated between laughing and crying. We knew it was what Connie would have wanted.

Case #12

KEPT AT ARM'S LENGTH

After the long relationship with my last case (Connie), I took an eight-week sabbatical from hospice in order to work through my grief. When a friend of my youngest daughter mentioned that her mother-in-law had entered hospice services, I requested the opportunity to be this woman's volunteer. The next day I was assigned to her (Mrs. Edwards) and given a brief oral summary of her illness.

Mrs. Edwards suffered from ovarian cancer, which had metastasized throughout her body. Her primary caretaker was her husband, who didn't want any "strangers in the house," although he had made a concession for the hospice nurse! He allowed their daughter-in-law to come in daily to bathe and dress Mrs. Edwards, who had wanted to remain as functional as possible. I phoned the daughter-in-law who said that Mrs. Edwards had declined to the point where she spent most of her time in bed. I asked that her father-in-law be told the hospice volunteer (me) would call in three days to see how she could be of assistance to the family.

When I did phone the husband, we had a pleasant 10-minute conversation; however, he insisted that "all bases were covered" and no help was needed. In fact, towards the end of the call, he became irate when telling me that five people had been in his house earlier in the day, upsetting both him and his wife. Apparently, the five people had been the hospice nurse, an aide, a nursing assistant, the daughter-in-law, and a neighbor bringing food. He said I could phone but I couldn't come over. I urged him to call me if he had any questions or if he wanted to share his feelings. He assured me that he would not!

When I called the following Monday morning, I again spoke with Mr. Edwards. He said his wife was exactly the same as the previous week, except for a leg neuropathy pain, which was worse than the cancer pain. I knew the hospice nurse was scheduled for a 1 p.m. visit so I encouraged him to discuss the issue of pain control with her. When I asked if I could bring them some food, he said that neighbors were bringing food and family members were picking up prescriptions. I then inquired as to whether he'd like a visit from the hospice spiritual counselor, but Mr. Edwards said they were members of the Roman Catholic Church. He added that their priest had made an unannounced visit the previous day, but he didn't let him in as his wife had already been given last rites when she was in the hospital!

The following Sunday, Mr. Edwards said his wife's leg pain seemed better, although she "bore pain well," so he wasn't really sure. He mentioned that she slept more and had weird, vivid dreams, although when awake, she had a clear mind and recognized family members. He again declined my offer to visit.

I waited seven days before my next phone call. At the time, Mr. Edwards was very abrupt with me and said that there had been no change and the weekend had gone well. He asked me not to call again until after Thanksgiving.

I called the Tuesday after Thanksgiving, and Mr. Edwards seemed more talkative. He said his wife had gone into a coma-like state and did not respond verbally nor open her eyes. I heard anxiousness in his voice. He said a home health aide had already been in the house for two hours, and he hoped that bathing his wife would make Mrs. Edwards feel better. I encouraged him to continue talking to his wife and assured him that the sense of hearing was the last to go. He sounded somewhat lost by not being able to communicate directly with her.

Four days later, I received word that Mrs. Edwards had died. I sent the family a sympathy card to express my condolences but, like my phone calls, it didn't seem enough.

Case #13

PREEMPTED

It was the first of the New Year when I was assigned to Mr. Hess, an 85- year-old gentleman with colon cancer, a colostomy, chronic heart failure, dementia, and pneumonia. He had been admitted to hospice the previous day, and started on Ativan for restlessness. I talked to his wife by phone who I mistook for his daughter due to her youthful voice. We set up an appointment for a next day "meet and greet" visit as I was eager to get involved.

Just before leaving home for this first visit with Mr. Hess, the hospice volunteer coordinator phoned to inform me that the family had requested a certain hospice volunteer they personally knew who lived in their town; so, I was taken off the case before I got started! I guess case #13 just wasn't a lucky one for me.

Case #14

THE GIFT

Two months passed before my next assignment, a 56-year-old woman named Jane. She had amyotrophic lateral sclerosis, sometimes referred to as "Lou Gehrig's disease." A dear aunt of mine had died from ALS, so I felt an immediate empathy.

Jane's adult son Kevin answered the phone when I called their house. When I explained that I was the assigned Hospice volunteer, he passed the phone to Jane. Her speech was slow and halting but welcoming. We arranged for me to visit at 1 p.m. the following Monday, a time when Jane's husband could be home to meet with me.

On Monday, I walked to their home which was nearby. It was snowing and everything looked pristine. Kevin greeted me at the door, saying that his work schedule consisted of random shifts, so he might be home occasionally. Jane sat on a wrap-around couch in their small living room. She looked much, much younger than her actual years, almost pixyish.

"The first thing to go was my vocal cords," she offered in a gravelly voice. Jane was, however, able to keep up her end of the conversation in a slow, low tone. She said she spent most of her days in her new electric wheelchair, and that an automated chair lift had recently been installed on the stairs to allow her to get upstairs to bed. We talked about the Hospice program, her special needs, and what I could offer as her volunteer. She seemed upbeat, resigned to her condition, and had no difficulty describing the onset of her disease to me, which had started with a toe drop and leg weakness. The actual diagnosis wasn't made until she exhibited multiple symptoms and went through three years of exhaustive testing.

Jane's husband, Jack, arrived home just before the end of my visit.

I must admit that he scared me at first. He had an extremely deep, intimidating voice and barked numerous questions at me to the point where I felt like I was being interrogated. When he was reassured that I was "okay," he abruptly went back to work. That's when Jane told me that he worked as a corrections officer locally and felt the need to "check me out."

On my next visit, both Jack and Kevin were

working, but each popped in once to check on Jane while I was with her. A scheduled speech therapist stopped by with a communication board, a specially designed laptop computer for the handicapped. As the therapist was late for another appointment, she rushed through the presentation, saying that if Jane didn't understand something, she could reference the manual. I tried to take notes but after the therapist left, both Jane and I felt overwhelmed and confused. Jane asked me to remove the laptop from her legs, and I was surprised at its heavy weight as I lifted it off her. Using the "joystick" (a hard, plastic thumb-shaped device) took dexterity and quick reaction times, which was impossible as Jane's right hand grew weaker each day. To complicate matters, her left hand was flaccid, as were her legs. We both agreed that the communication board was a fiasco. Meanwhile, Jane said she had a bladder infection, which had been detected the previous day on a routine doctor's visit. Unfortunately, the medicine the doctor had prescribed for the infection made her nauseous.

A 26-inch snowfall prevented my next appointment so we rescheduled. When I showed up at 1 p.m. the following day, Jane was visibly upset. An older hospice volunteer was with her who, according to Jane, "wouldn't leave." Son Kevin had arrived home from work a half hour earlier and had told the volunteer she could leave but, for some reason, the lady didn't know what to do. She had called the hospice office to request that a social worker be sent out. Jane was crying in frustration because she didn't want the social worker to come. Sizing up the situation, I convinced the elderly volunteer that I would take over, and then I phoned the office to cancel the social worker. I attempted to soothe Jane and apologize for the confusion. Jane was a very bright woman who could think clearly. She was definitely capable of making her own decisions but, as she pointed out, due to her physical deterioration from ALS, people didn't always listen to her. Jane emphatically verbalized to me that she wanted no visitors unless they first made an appointment. I told her I would let the hospice office know her policy. We were then able to relax together and spend an hour talking about our favorite books and movies.

With Jane's permission, I visited on Mondays and Fridays. One day, we talked about music and I sang for her. Jane said she wished she had a piano so I could play for her also. She said her favorite hymn was "Victory in Jesus," one I had never heard. Toward the end of the visit, I gave Jane a copy of my favorite novel *The Secret Life of Bees*, as reading was a pastime she still enjoyed. Jane said she would read it and report back! Some of her church friends arrived just before I left.

There was a snowfall before my next visit, but I was able to walk to Jane's house as planned. She was talkative and had read some of the novel I had lent her. While taking a sip of water, however, she choked and had trouble getting her breathing synchronized. Her cough reflex was feeble. She tried to blow her nose but could not. She had no abdominal muscle strength to push any air. She seemed thinner on this visit. A church friend stopped by for the last half hour I was there.

What a fun time we had on the following visit. Jane's husband and son were both at work so we were totally alone. The vacuum cleaner was lying on the living room floor as usual since Jane had never let me move it. Today I explained how much I loved cleaning, organizing, and straightening, and how I wished she'd let me help her in this way. She surprised me by agreeing. When I finished, she wheeled out to the kitchen to inspect my work. She was delighted to see the kitchen counter clean, the dishes put away, and the floor spotless. She said she had prided herself on always keeping a clean house and wished she could still do so. Under her direction, I made her half a sandwich, but she could only manage a few bites. She again choked on her water. I wondered how much longer she'd be able to eat solid foods.

Jane was on the couch when I next arrived and was decidedly irritated. The source of her bad mood was a large oxygen tank, tubing, and suction equipment lying in the middle of the living room. According to her, she didn't want it, hadn't asked for it, and wanted it gone. I could only surmise that the hospice nurse who oversaw Jane's progress must have felt that the oxygen machine was necessary. Jane made it clear to me that she wanted no artificial intervention, and this included oxygen. In addition, she said that if she ever choked, she did not want the Heimlich maneuver. She emphatically stated that if she choked to death, "so be it." These statements made me feel very uncomfortable, and I urged her to talk with her hospice nurse. As Jane calmed down, we discussed books, and she said she really had enjoyed *The Secret Life of Bees*, especially the nurturing relationship between the older women and the young girl. Later in our visit, she allowed me to scrub the half bath and wash the kitchen floor. Then we sat together and looked through her hymnal. She chose five hymns she wanted played at her funeral. They were: "Victory in Jesus," "To God Be the Glory," "Jesus Saves," "Amazing Grace," and "How Great Thou Art." She lent me the hymnal so I could practice the first three hymns on my piano at home, as I was unfamiliar with them. I hoped to be able to sing them a cappella to her if I could grasp the melodies and rhythms.

A week went by and on our next visit, I could

not get in the door! Both locks were on, and Jane was home alone. She and I yelled back and forth to one another from opposite sides of the front door. She managed to turn the bottom lock but wasn't strong enough to unlock the deadbolt. With quick problem-solving skills, Jane phoned a church friend who had an extra key. I then walked two blocks to the church day care center where the friend worked, retrieved the key and was able to enter the house. The first thing I noticed was the oxygen equipment still lying on the floor but, because Jane was ignoring it, so did I. We listened to the hymns I had recorded onto a cassette tape. Jane, who was Baptist, laughed and said I was playing "Victory in Jesus" much too slowly. I laughed and said it was probably due to my Episcopal upbringing!

A few days later, an occupational therapist was leaving as I arrived. The OT had brought foam to make a larger grip area on Jane's utensils. Jane shook her head in disgust as she showed me that the actual utensils were too large to push through the hole in the foam. She decided she didn't want the OT to come back. On this visit, Jane didn't want me doing any housework so we talked about religious experiences. We both felt safe enough with each other to share personal stories about angels. I left when the Hospice nurse arrived but not before hearing her explain to Jane that the oxygen equipment was remaining in the home at her husband's request. Jane then agreed.

A friend of Jane's was chatting with her when I arrived for my next scheduled visit. I had brought a CD with me entitled "It's Hard to See Jesus," which had been recorded by a local Hospice nurse. It surprised me when Jane said she didn't like the lyrics. She said that for her, it was easy to see Jesus! Today I sensed that Jane had made a downward turn in her health, but I couldn't cite anything specific.

When I arrived for my next visit, I was greeted by Sylvia, a woman Jane's husband had hired to stay with her when he and his son were both at work. Jack trusted Sylvia as she was also in law enforcement and was doing this as a favor and a side job. Jane was wearing a neck brace she got from the ALS clinic the day before. There was also an additional wheelchair strap holding down her left leg, which had been jumpy. A pillow was wedged between her knees as they occasionally knocked together. Jane said her "good" hand, the right one, was starting to weaken, and I noticed that her speech was more slurred, making it harder for her to produce words. Sylvia helped transfer her to and from the toilet, and Jane was pleased that she still had control of her bodily functions.

On my next visit, Jane and I had some time alone as Sylvia left when I arrived. I shared some family stories that Jane found amusing. On another visit, I took a bicycle horn with me. I felt Jane might want it in order to summon help as she could no longer yell. She laughingly declined, showing me a button on her electric wheelchair that beeped outrageously loud (it scared me when she pushed it). When she blew that horn, I realized I needed to ask before assuming a need.

I had to share my next visit with Jane's church friend who stopped by while I was there. The lady seemed determined to make sure I was "saved" and even insisted I take a pamphlet home to read. Jane seemed depressed because she could no longer read; she couldn't hold a book or turn pages. I asked if she'd allow me to read to her, but she flatly refused.

On a subsequent visit, I asked Jane why she wouldn't allow me to read to her. Through hand gestures, she made me understand that she couldn't absorb the gist of a story when it was read aloud and that was why she didn't listen to book tapes. She then pointed outdoors, and I agreed that it was a gloriously sunny warm spring day. I asked if there was any way she could go outside, and she quickly maneuvered her wheelchair into the kitchen. I joked with her that she could enter the wheelchair Olympics because, even with her weak right hand, she could get the chair to do what she wanted. She had me place a block of wood (custom-made by her son) at the bottom of the kitchen door-sill so she could use it as a ramp to get through the door onto the back deck. I sat in a patio chair next to her on the deck while we watched neighborhood children play. We listened to the birds sing while the sun's rays warmed us both.

Two weeks passed before I saw Jane again as her son canceled one of my scheduled visits. I learned that she'd had Easter dinner with her husband's relatives. There had been a huge family gathering, and she had enjoyed seeing everyone and being out in the spring weather.

Jane's wheelchair was tilted back at a steep angle when I arrived the next time. Caregiver Sylvia told me that Jane could no longer sit upright as she would fall forward. When Sylvia transferred Jane from the wheelchair to the couch, it looked like she was dancing with a lifesized rag doll. Once seated, Jane's socks pooled at her ankles since her legs were like sticks.

Kevin, her son, was home with Jane on my next visit. The three of us sat and watched CSNBC with Jane being surprisingly aloof. I felt unwelcome. When I told her I'd be on vacation for the next two weeks, she didn't respond.

When I returned from vacation, Jane could only moan and use crude body language. I told her about my Florida trip and, unlike the previous visit, she seemed pleased to be with me.

On my last attempt to see Jane for a scheduled visit, I walked to her home in the rain only to be turned away by her son, who finally answered the doorbell on the third pronounced ring. He said his mother chose to stay in bed and that he had canceled the Hospice nurse but had forgotten to call me. When I asked if I could just sit quietly with Jane, Kevin said no. He did say I could visit the following week. I walked home disappointed.

Two days after this attempted visit, Jane died. Sadly, I attended an evening funeral viewing and service. Her casket was closed but there was a memory board of photos nearby. The family's church pastor led a 45-minute service, which included the singing of Jane's five favorite hymns. Afterwards, I had a chance to talk to Jane's son and tell him how much I admired the care he had given her. I mentioned how he had understood her slurred speech and attempts at communication when no one else could.

Just before leaving the funeral home, Jane's husband, Jack, greeted me by saying that I was one of the few people Jane had let visit her. He said she always looked forward to my visits. (I never knew this.) Jack said that during the afternoon viewing, the piano cassette I had made for Jane had played continuously and he thanked me for it. Jack didn't realize it, but he had just given me a gift from Jane.

Case #15

JUST ANOTHER LIFE EXPERIENCE

It had been two months since my last case, so when the hospice volunteer coordinator called to assign me as the primary volunteer to an 82-year-old gentleman named Arthur who suffered from colon, bladder, and liver cancer, I was happy to be needed again. I was told the wife wanted someone to stay with her husband at 2 p.m. that afternoon so she could get her hair done. Unfortunately, I had another obligation, but I was able to make arrangements to arrive at 1 p.m. and have another volunteer relieve me at 2 p.m.

I was met at the door by the man's youngest daughter, Wilma. The house was a small rancher with two bedrooms directly off the living/dining area. There was a lot of activity both outside and inside the house as the client owned a home-based trucking business, which his oldest son had taken over. Four of the couple's five grown children lived in the immediate area and were continually stopping by.

Wilma introduced me to Arthur's wife, Winona, who had a very youthful appearance and energetic way of speaking. We sat and talked at the dining room table, the central meeting place for the family. I explained that this was a meet-and-greet visit so that we could determine where I could help out as their regular volunteer. I learned that the patient, Arthur, had been a volunteer fireman for thirty years, eventually becoming the fire chief. While talking, phone and doorbell interruptions were many. Another daughter joined us at the table and stated that her father kept saying he needed a ticket to "get on the bus." He would also ask for his shoes. I shared that those statements often indicated that the patient was getting ready to take a journey (in this case his final transition), which was being conveyed in a type of verbal sign language. I encouraged her to talk about some of her fondest memories of family life with her father whenever she was at his bedside.

Winona then took me into their bedroom to meet Arthur, who was lying in a hospital bed facing a wall. The head of his bed was at the foot of his wife's bed, creating an L-shape. Hanging on the wall directly in Arthur's line of vision was an old work calendar from 1931. Winona left us alone to talk. After introducing myself, I told Arthur that my father-in-law had been a volunteer fireman. Arthur talked about his own volunteer firefighter experiences, although loud voices from the dining room were distracting, often causing Arthur to stop and look around. On one occasion, he pointed to the wall he faced and asked me to open a box and retrieve an item. There was no box. I redirected our conversation and wished I could stay with him longer but at 1:45, the substitute hospice volunteer relieved me so that his wife could leave for her appointment. Before I left the house, I made arrangements with Winona to visit again in two days.

On the way home, I thought about things I could discuss with Winona that might help Arthur have a more pleasant passing, such as turning his bed around so that he faced the bedroom window. Also, I could suggest they remove the confusing 1931 calendar and put up some family photos instead.

The next day, Winona left a message on my answering machine saying she didn't need me to come out on Thursday and that she'd be in touch. I returned her call to reschedule my next visit but she bluntly refused, indicating that she wanted to spend more time at Arthur's bedside. She added that she didn't need any more distractions. I asked if I could phone the following week, and she emphatically said no in a very dismissive tone, saying that if she needed me, she'd call but not to call her. On this note, my rosy plans for Arthur flew out the window.

Ten days later, the hospice volunteer coordinator called to say that Arthur had died. I mentally reviewed the situation to see what I might have done differently. Maybe I talked too much on that first visit and didn't listen enough; maybe Winona only needed a one-time babysitter; or maybe, it was just another life experience.

Case #16

CD SEND-OFF

I was assigned the next patient because she lived in the cul-de-sac across the street from me, although I had never met the family before. Geraldine charmed me the moment I met her, so it was a shame I only had the chance to visit with her twice.

On our first encounter, she was alert and appeared to understand that I was a hospice volunteer as well as her neighbor. She had lived with her son and daughter-in-law for a few years. Her bedroom was a lovely peach color with large windows next to her hospital bed. She had fuzzy cropped white hair, the result of chemotherapy following a hysterectomy for uterine cancer. Unfortunately, the cancer had metastasized to her brain.

Geraldine was watching an old-time movie during my first visit and, at times, she would intertwine the movie plot with real life before snapping back to reality. After introducing myself to her, I sat in a rocker next to her bed so we could talk in-between TV/mental excursions. A round table to the left of her bed held many angel figurines as well as a statue of the Blessed Virgin Mary. Geraldine told me she was a very devout Roman Catholic. I shared that I was an Episcopalian and also an angel collector, and that I would bring my favorite angel to show her on our next visit. After 15 minutes of pleasant conversation, she began calling loudly for her adult son, George, her primary caretaker. When he entered the room, I quietly walked down the stairs to give them privacy although I heard her say to George, "I don't know who that woman is but she wouldn't leave!"

I had arranged to visit two days later but George called and cancelled the visit. He said his mother was sleeping all the time, and I wasn't needed. It gave us a chance to talk about other services I could provide, such as light housekeeping, making meals, gardening, etc., but he wasn't comfortable with those options. A few days later, I brought the family some homemade zucchini bread and zucchini lasagna because our garden had produced zucchinis faster than I could keep up. George's wife called the next day to thank me, and we had a nice chat about her mother-in-law.

I sat with Geraldine a week later as George

needed to run some errands. She slept the entire time. The TV was on a religious channel but the sound had been muted. The family had set up a CD player on the dresser, which played classical music. George said they only had two CDs, and he needed to get more. I offered him a CD I brought with me on home visits entitled *Classical Healing* and urged him to keep it as long as needed. I stayed for an hour-long bedside vigil that day.

Geraldine died three days after my second visit. Due to prior commitments, I couldn't attend her viewing, but I was able to go to her funeral, which was held on a Thursday morning at 10:30. The funeral was held in a town unfamiliar to me, and I had to take two busy beltways to get there. The exit ramp I needed to take was just beyond a large construction area. Unfortunately, I was in the wrong lane and missed my ramp. I got off at the next exit, totally lost. Sign choices indicated "Baltimore" or "Washington," but due to impatient drivers blowing their horns behind me, I took a small access road which unexpectedly ended up in the town I needed! After flagging down a Federal Express truck, the driver gave me excellent directions and I arrived at the church one minute before the funeral mass began. I truly believe that angels must have led me to the church.

These same angels must have been off-duty for the ride home as I made a wrong choice and ended up in the Ft. McHenry tunnel headed in the opposite direction from what I needed. Thankfully, a pleasant toll taker gave me directions that eventually led me home after a two hour unnecessary detour.

A week later, George returned my classical CD. He said his mother had remained very peaceful when it played, so they had left it on 24/7. He shared that the CD had been playing when she died, news that I found very comforting.

Case #17

EVERYONE PLEASE LEAVE

For this case, I was asked to drive 20 miles from home to see an elderly woman named Cynthia, who resided in an upscale nursing home. The volunteer coordinator said the woman loved hymns, so I could sing to her. She said that the patient's daughter, Jackie, who resided on the West Coast, was temporarily staying in the room with her mother. Apparently, Cynthia had a fast growing kidney cancer, and the family was very anxious. They had requested daily nursing visits from hospice and any other services that could be provided, including a volunteer.

My first visit to the patient was chaotic. Cynthia was lying on her side, asleep in a hospital bed in a surprisingly small, crowded room. Her mouth was agape and her breathing was loud. The blinds in the room were shut tightly, and everyone was whispering. The daughter who was supposed to be in the room was not there; instead, Cynthia's three large grown granddaughters hovered in a tiny space at the head of her bed. The patient's son, a tall tired-looking man, stood nearby. When I explained that I was Cynthia's hospice volunteer, it took him a few moments to digest the information before responding. I introduced myself again, and the gentleman told me his name was Ben and then asked me to "kindly wait down the hall."

There were two chairs at the end of the hallway where I went to sit. Five minutes passed before Ben and a beautiful, stately older woman approached me. The elderly woman was dressed impeccably. She walked with a gorgeous gold inlay wooden cane and sat in the chair next to mine while Ben stood. She introduced herself as Aunt Mamie, sister of the patient. She queried, "What exactly do you do, dear?" I explained my hospice volunteer status and that I had been told that Cynthia loved hymns, so I wanted to sing to her. Aunt Mamie nodded encouragingly. I suggested that the family might like to have lunch in the cafeteria while I spent time alone with their loved one. Definitely in charge, Aunt Mamie agreed. She herded her nephew and three grandnieces to the cafeteria but not before telling me that the patient's daughter, who had been staying with Cynthia, had returned to California.

When I re-entered Cynthia's room, she seemed fitful and in pain. Her body was rigidly curled in a fetal position. I placed a small pillow between her knees, which seemed to ease her distress somewhat. After opening the blinds to get enough light to see the words in my hymnal, I began singing softly. Unfortunately, our quiet time together didn't last long. Interruptions were constant. A woman entered the room who said she had been a companion to "Miz Cynthia" when Cynthia had been well. This same woman began sobbing loudly and blowing her nose while leaning over the bed to tell me about her personal life. With as much tact as possible, I guided her from the room and suggested she might want to return at a later date.

When I began singing to Cynthia again, there was more knocking at the door. In walked an elderly candy-striper pushing a woman in a wheelchair. The wheelchair woman, Lavinia, was yet another sister of the patient who also lived in this same facility. The striper explained that Lavinia wanted to see her sister and listen to me sing. As I started singing, the aide yanked Cynthia's hand toward Lavinia in an attempt to have them hold hands. Immediately, Cynthia cried out in pain and the striper apologized profusely. As politely as possible, I suggested they also might want to come back at another time. Thankfully, they left.

I stroked Cynthia's forehead while singing, and
she drifted back to sleep. Shortly thereafter, a
staff nurse came in to administer a dropper of pain
medication, followed by two other staff members
"just checking." Hymns were peppered around
this never-ending activity.

When Aunt Mamie, Ben, and the three grandchildren returned, I gave them a copy of a classical
healing CD and suggested that someone bring in
a CD player and let the music play lightly in the
background. I explained how the last sense to go
was hearing and that sometimes soothing music
could help a patient make the transition peacefully.
I encouraged each of them to lean over the bed
and share a favorite memory with her. I agreed to
return in three days.

Only one person was with Cynthia on my next
visit—the daughter, Jackie, who obviously had not
returned to her home in California. She appeared
to be a no-nonsense woman as she paced ner-
vously by the bedside. She carried on a loud con-
tinuous one-way conversation with her mother but
Cynthia neither opened her eyes nor responded
verbally.

I was pleased to note that the hospice nurse
had gotten the patient's pain under control as she
was no longer restless or posturing on this visit.
Cynthia's coloring was a lovely pink, and she was
lying comfortably on her back. Her mouth was

wide open, and her breaths were deep, coming at long intervals of 20 seconds apart. I checked the bag draped from the bed rail and noted that Cynthia's urine was clear. It didn't look like she was in any hurry to depart. A new CD player sat on the bedside table. Jackie said her brother Ben had told her about me, and then she rattled off a long list of her mother's favorite hymns. In the midst of this recitation, Ben arrived and emphatically told Jackie that I knew what I was doing. *Uh-oh,* I thought. When I began singing my first hymn, Jackie surprised me by joining in. I don't think I've ever heard anyone sing totally off-key for an entire song before; the effect was absolutely jarring. To my relief, Ben stood up abruptly, told Jackie they were going to the cafeteria, and whisked her out of the room.

After their departure, I actually spent an entire hour alone with the patient and was able to sing without interruption before the hospice nurse, Mimi, walked into the room. She said that Cynthia couldn't last much longer with such large intervals between breaths; however, her circulation was still good and there was no fluid in her lungs.

Mimi shared that Cynthia was the oldest of five sisters and had been the matriarch of the family. Obviously, she intended to die when she wanted to and not on anyone else's timetable. I shared my feeling that the patient was never left alone long enough to have the quietude necessary to make the transition. Mimi agreed, and said she'd talk to the family about our concerns. As if on cue, Ben and Jackie returned. Mimi went out into the hallway to speak with them while I sang a few closing hymns before turning on the classical healing CD. I said my goodbyes to the family and promised to return at the same time in three days.

Three days later as I prepared to visit Cynthia, I was notified that she had died peacefully the previous night. I couldn't help but wonder how she had managed to slip away.

Case #18

JUST KEEP READING

After Ms. Cynthia died, I took a few months off before accepting my next patient, Sarah. She had entered the hospice program three months earlier, but at that time, Sarah had refused volunteer services. Now the family needed volunteer help, and I lived in close proximity. Had we been destined to connect?

Teri (one of the patient's adult daughters) and her husband had moved into Sarah's home once treatment options had ceased for her. They brought their three horses, one dog, and two cats to add to the animal population already living in this farmhouse setting.

Sarah and I met for the first time upstairs in the bedroom she shared with her husband, Jeff. A hospital bed had been pushed up against their four-poster double bed so that husband and wife could remain sleeping next to each other at night. Daughter Teri had let me into the house and had brought me upstairs to meet Sarah. Teri then crawled into the double bed next to her mother as Teri was pregnant and suffering from morning sickness.

Sarah and I took to each other instantly. She explained that 18 years earlier, she'd had a cancerous mole (melanoma) removed from her left forearm. Because the doctors felt they had gotten it all, no other treatment was performed at that time. However, this past summer when Sarah had trouble breathing, it was discovered that the melanoma had metastasized throughout her lungs and body. Subsequently, she underwent aggressive chemotherapy unsuccessfully. One of Sarah's sisters, a Hospice nurse who lived in another state, had urged her to enter our local Hospice program which she did.

Although I asked how I could be of service to Sarah and Teri, neither of them could think of anything. I suggested that I might visit twice a week for a couple hours at a time so Teri could go outside for fresh air. Because I had noticed an upright piano downstairs, I told them I was a piano teacher and would be glad to play any of their favorite pieces, which seemed agreeable to them. Subsequently, whenever my visits coincided with an aide giving Sarah a bath, I would retreat to the piano to play classical music or hymns.

One afternoon, I noticed a novel sitting on Sarah's bedside table and remarked that it was my favorite book. Sarah said the book had been given to her by a friend who knew she loved reading but that nowadays, she couldn't concentrate enough to read. I asked if I could read the book to her out loud during my visits. Sarah agreed. On this same visit, Sarah told me all about her wonderful hospice nurse with whom she had developed a special bond. Apparently, the nurse had given Sarah several funny, heart-warming videos that both she and her daughter enjoyed watching from the side-by-side beds. "Entertainment for the sickies," commented Sarah.

One of Sarah's out-of-town sisters came the following week to cook, clean, and visit, so I was asked to keep in touch by telephone only. Two weeks after my initial contact, I visited again. Although a pregnant Teri didn't feel well enough to go outdoors, she went into another bedroom to work on a scrap-booking project while I spent time alone with Sarah. I was impressed with the large dry erase message board that Teri had hung on Sarah's bedroom door, directly across from her bed.

In bold, large black letters, it listed the 7 days of the week, specifying the month and date. In columns beneath each day, Teri had written the names of people who would be visiting and the time of day they were coming. At the very bottom of the board, each hospice caregiver's full name and phone number was listed. I could see that it gave Sarah a sense of control over the daily happenings.

Sarah looked good to me. Although catheterized, she said she was performing physical therapy exercises each day to strengthen her legs so she could eventually walk to the bathroom with the use of a cane. Her goal was to get strong enough to go downstairs to the kitchen and cook the family meals again. After mutual sharing and talking, we agreed that I'd begin reading to her on my next visit.

Unfortunately, my next visit was cancelled as Sarah had fallen. She hadn't broken anything but, according to Teri, Sarah was bruised all over. Physical therapy on her legs had to be discontinued as her legs weren't strong enough to withstand the exercises. When I finally did visit, Sarah said the hardest part after the fall was climbing back into bed knowing it was where she would have to remain. The loss of hope in her voice was difficult to hear. I started reading the book out loud but she soon fell asleep.

The next time we saw each other, Sarah asked that I begin reading the novel again and said she'd try her best not to fall asleep! We stopped after three chapters when Sarah tired. She was pleased that she could keep track of the characters, saying she was eager to hear the rest of the story. Before leaving the house, I noticed that her ankles were swollen.

When we next met, daughter Teri drove to the library for a few hours, leaving us alone. Sarah boasted that I was lucky to find her alive because the previous night, she had experienced excruciating leg pain. Her left leg had swelled up and turned blue. Morphine hadn't helped. She said the pain was similar to what she had experienced in her lung a few months earlier when a metastatic tumor had caused a blood clot. She said her husband Jeff had remained awake the entire night, scared that he might lose her. She said she had "walked through the valley of the shadow of death" and had faced her fears. She said she realized now that others had gone before her and that when she did die, she would be okay. Needless to say, we didn't do any reading.

On my next visit, I read several chapters aloud and Sarah got very caught up in the action. Her husband stopped by to say hello when he had a break in his work activities. It was nice to meet him as Sarah had spoken so lovingly about him.

The next time I saw Sarah, we read one particularly difficult chapter in the novel in which the main character, a teenage girl, gets beaten by her father. I had to stop and reach for a Kleenex. Sarah motioned to have the box passed to her and we both dabbed our eyes. She then began talking about her first husband who was "just as mean," which led to more sharing of her personal life. The book seemed to release a flood of memories for her. She shared that she had gotten out of a bad first marriage and made it on her own for the sake of her children. Sarah also said how blessed she felt to have such a loving husband now. We cried many times that day while reading and each time we did, Sarah related another chapter of her own life. The book was an amazing catalyst. Before leaving though, I noticed there was blood in Sarah's urine bag.

On a subsequent visit, the novel described a funeral held for one of the characters. Sarah mentioned that while undergoing chemotherapy, she had put her will in order and her funeral wishes on paper. She said she had also written something for each of her daughters that would be given to them after she died. She said that her family was scattered "around the country" and that they'd probably gather for a picnic remembrance, which was what she wanted. She said, "Life should be about fun," and she hoped they'd share funny stories about her.

Although Sarah's daughter cancelled my next visit, with her permission, I stopped by with some homemade soup and pumpernickel bread. Teri said that a large tumor had popped out on Sarah's right side and one was pressing on her neck. According to Teri, Sarah seemed more tired and was having trouble keeping track of things. Thankfully, the following week when I visited, Sarah managed to follow the story line in our book. We agreed, after another mutual crying jag, that this book had a powerful cathartic effect on both of us, letting emotionally painful areas well up and be released. We were 40 pages away from completing the book when I left that day, and Sarah was feeling a sense of urgency to finish it.

On my next visit, I met Sarah's other daughter who had come to visit, as well as her husband. Also congregated in the house were Sarah's two sisters and their husbands who had recently arrived. Despite all the company, Sarah was adamant that we finish the book *today.* Family members agreed to let us have time together and were kind enough to stay downstairs.

A half hour into our reading, a substitute nurse's aide arrived unexpectedly to give Sarah a bath. As I got up to leave the room, Sarah insisted that I sit back down and continue reading while she got bathed. Sarah was naked from the waist up and was lying on her side when we reached another sad section in the book. She lunged for the nearest pillow to bury her face to sop up her tears but in doing so, Sarah's tumor-ridden body got stuck in the crease between the two beds! At the aide's request, I crawled up on the larger bed and pushed on Sarah's bare shoulders while the aide pulled from the other side. Sarah started laughing hysterically. She made jokes about her flopping breasts while the aide and I played "heave-ho." We finally got Sarah turned over but the three of us couldn't stop laughing for quite some time.

After the aide left, Sarah and I finished reading another chapter when the hospice nurse arrived unannounced. The small 10x12 bedroom was already over-crowded with a hospital bed, adjoining double bed, dresser, bedside commode, bedside table, and rocking chair, not to mention three people and now the dog that had pushed open the door. I must say, nothing in my hospice training had covered this type of situation. However, it *was* funny and faintly reminiscent of a Marx brother's movie. Sarah insisted I keep reading while the nurse checked her vitals and, believe it or not, we managed to finish the book and have a final laugh and cry together before I left.

Teri cancelled my next visit, saying Sarah was exhausted from all the company. The following week when I did visit, I started reading aloud a new novel but Sarah slept through the entire visit. Her husband was home at the time and said she had been sleeping a lot and when awake, she was disoriented. I intended to see Sarah again the following Tuesday.

My next visit was cancelled by a family member who phoned to say Sarah had passed away. When I later talked to daughter Teri, she said Sarah had passed away quietly in her sleep. At Sarah's request, her body was donated to science and there was no funeral. I hoped that the family would eventually hold the remembrance picnic, replete with funny stories, as Sarah had wanted.

Case #19

FIRED AND HURTING

Four weeks after Sarah died, I was assigned a new patient, Agnes. She was the same age as my mother and suffered from the same disease of emphysema. I wondered if there would be parallels in their process or outcome.

I spoke with Selma, Agnes's daughter-in-law, by phone the night before my first visit. Agnes lived with her eldest son and his wife, Selma. When Agnes was admitted to hospice, Selma took a three-month leave-of-absence from her job to become the primary caregiver.

On my initial visit, Selma met me at the door and walked me to the upstairs bedroom where Agnes lay in a hospital bed. The small room was painted a cheerful color and had a window and small television. I wasn't expecting to see a patient so robust and talkative. Agnes quickly informed me that Selma was a "daughter" to her in every way and that the word "in-law" was taboo. Agnes went on to tell me about her own wonderful marriage, the shock of her husband's unexpected death this past Easter, and how awful she felt at being a burden to her two sons.

She verbalized that she'd "rather be dead than need to have someone wipe my behind." As I was leaving, Selma motioned me into the kitchen where we couldn't be overheard. She cried and said she loved Agnes very much and wanted to do everything possible for her, but she was exhausted from lack of sleep. I encouraged Selma to let me visit often, even if it was just so that she could nap.

I was supposed to visit on Monday but Selma called to say Agnes's other daughter-in-law had taken off from work that day and wanted to spend time alone with her. Selma went on to say that Agnes was in a foul mood because the hospice nurse had informed her that she had made improvement since entering hospice. (Once a patient's medications are regulated for good pain control and medical management, there is often an improvement in their condition.) Apparently for Agnes, who wanted to join her deceased husband, this was not welcome news.

A week later, I stayed with Agnes while Selma ran errands. For 90 minutes, Agnes talked about her life, her children, and her marriage. Although this dialog was pleasant, I could see by the frown at her brow that she was troubled. I asked if she had any concerns. She said her bowels weren't moving, and the nurse had suggested that Selma administer a suppository to her that evening. Agnes found the thought humiliating and said, "I don't know what I've done to deserve this—Why me?" Out of my mouth popped, "Why not?" Agnes looked at me with a stunned expression on her face. I quickly explained that I had just finished reading a book about the dying process which had helped me resolve some of my own emotional issues and that one of the phrases in the book to questions like "Why me?" was "Why not?"

In retrospect, I can see how very cold and harsh my comment may have seemed to Agnes that day. I said I'd love to bring the book along on my next visit and read some of it to her but Agnes said she didn't see how any book could help her understand her situation any better. I asked her to think about it, and she responded, "I don't need one more thing to think about." Selma came home at that moment, and we agreed that I would return the following Tuesday so that Selma could have some time off.

As I hadn't heard from Selma by Monday, I phoned her that evening. Selma said that the other daughter-in-law would be staying with Agnes on Tuesday and that she'd call me if and when she needed me.

The following morning, my hospice supervisor called to tell me that the family had requested that I be removed from the case. Apparently, the family had complained to the hospice social worker about my insensitivity, particularly about my insistence on reading a certain book to the patient. When I heard this, I felt like my insides collapsed. The truth of the situation hit me smack in the solar plexus. I felt ashamed and began doubting my ability to ever be a good hospice volunteer again, or for that matter, if ever I would be allowed to try again.

After two weeks of emotionally beating myself up and feeling very dark in my soul, I lit a candle in prayer. I poured my heart out to God, admitting that my enthusiasm and good intentions had run away with me. I had fallen back into an old habit of trying to control and direct the lives of others. In hospice, we are taught to "meet the patient where they are" and accompany them on their journey. We should let them lead us, not the opposite. I had another cry, asked God for forgiveness, and blew out the candle. I felt like a weight had been lifted from my shoulders.

Within an hour, the phone rang. It was my hospice supervisor asking me to take another case. "You mean you still believe in me?" I queried. She said we all make mistakes, and she was sure I had learned from this one. She encouraged me to let it go and move on. I moved on but never forgot the lesson. I hope I have honored Agnes by becoming a better hospice volunteer.

Case #20

THE PIANO

In June, I was assigned to Neil, a 53-year-old male with leukemia, who had always prided himself on being a "man's man." He had been a truck driver all his life, and had enjoyed hunting, fishing, and riding motorcycles. For four years prior to his diagnosis, Neil and partner Lucy had been living together happily.

The past February, after having been ill for several weeks, Neil was told he had leukemia. Chemotherapy was offered to delay the course of the disease, but the doctors said his only real chance for a full remission was a bone marrow transplant. Two of his siblings were too old to donate bone marrow, one sibling's blood didn't match, and one brother wouldn't consider becoming a donor due to a ten-year feud.

Chemotherapy began in March, and Neil had

blood work every two weeks to monitor for any changes. He was told each time that the disease was not progressing. In May, he and Lucy married but shortly thereafter, Neil began running a high fever which doctors attributed to a virus. When the fever continued for two additional weeks, he was sent to an infectious disease specialist. The specialist hospitalized him for a battery of tests. The initial blood work showed that Neil was in the final stages of leukemia. When the doctor told him he had less than a month to live, Neil became furious. He questioned how the disease could have "suddenly" gotten to end-stage. He was discharged home and reluctantly entered hospice care.

At Lucy's request when I was assigned to this case, I had only spoken to her by phone without actually visiting Neil. She had cried each time we talked on the phone as she was emotionally and physically exhausted. She said Neil remained in a rage. He refused any special equipment such as a hospital bed, which would have made things easier for both of them. According to her, Neil bellowed at her when she didn't bring items to him fast enough. She said she "knew it wasn't the real Neil talking, but it still hurt."

One day I received a phone call from the hospice nurse assigned to this case. She said she was calling from Neil's home and that Lucy was standing beside her. The nurse asked if I could visit the next day for two hours so that Lucy could take a nap. The way the nurse slowly formed her words made me realize how important it was that I show up, so I cleared my schedule.

It was chaotic when I arrived at their home the next day. The hospice nurse and a hospice aide were both there. Neil had refused to take any medicine that morning and had become very agitated. Although extremely weak, he had stumbled out of bed and fallen. Neil didn't break anything physically, but he was bruised and continued to fight anyone who tried to assist him. The nurse somehow managed to give him a shot to calm him. She then ordered a hospital bed, which arrived shortly after I did. Once Neil was settled in the hospital bed, the nurse came into the kitchen to speak with Lucy and me. She said Neil's platelet count was so low that there was a good chance he could "bleed out," proving fatal. She gathered old towels and gave them to the aide, who planned to stay at his bedside. The nurse told Lucy to get as much rest as possible since it looked like only a matter of one or two days before Neil would pass away. I was asked to handle the phones. The nurse left but said she'd be back later in the afternoon to install a morphine pump.

When Lucy went to a bedroom to lie down, I sat in the living room near the phone, which was next to a spinet piano. About an hour into my visit,

Lucy came out to say she was "too wired to sleep." She said she was going to Walmart to pick up a baby monitor for Neil's room. I asked if I could play the piano while she was gone, and she said "sure."

I never heard Lucy when she returned to the house. When I stopped playing the piano, Lucy came into the living room and said she had been home for a half hour. She asked if I could continue playing while she ate her lunch, as she found the music very soothing. She also said that it was the first time in days that she had felt calm. I played classical music for another hour, and Lucy gave me a big hug before I left. I was glad Lucy had found some peace, if only for a short time. Neil died the following morning.

Case #20.5

THE SUBSTITUTE

My best friend, Mary, is also a hospice volunteer. We met while taking hospice classes and immediately bonded like sisters. We often shared hospice experiences and suggestions with one another. When she was preparing to go on vacation, Mary asked if I'd look in on her patient, Carolyn, while she was gone. I said I'd be happy to do so.

Mary said that Carolyn lived in an assisted living private home setting, that she had dementia and was often confused although, at times, she could be quite coherent. So, I wasn't sure what to expect.

On my first visit, Carolyn was sitting on a couch in a cozy living room. Three other ladies sat around the perimeter of the same room in recliner chairs. As usual, I wore my large hospice name badge. I made it a point to sit down next to Carolyn on the sofa. She scowled at me when I told her my name was Linda and that I was substituting for Mary, her regular hospice volunteer. I told her Mary was on vacation but she would return on Monday. Carolyn looked intensely at me and then said, "You've gotten too skinny!" I couldn't help smiling and knew Mary would too when I told her that Carolyn had gotten us mixed up (Mary is short and round, and I am tall and thin!).

Carolyn and I sat together quietly on the couch for a few minutes longer before I tried some conversation starters, such as "Isn't it a beautiful day?" and "How long have you lived here?" To each question, she either responded "None of your business" or "That's for me to know." Even the other workers in the home were greeted with angry outbursts from her as they entered the room. I later found out that Carolyn had refused her medication and food all day, which may have had something to do with her foul mood. I didn't give up, though, and stayed with her for another half hour. This time I sat quietly, saying nothing. After a few minutes, Carolyn relaxed and snuggled up to me, laying her head on my shoulder.

I visited Carolyn again the next day, and she seemed like a different person. She was happy to see me as we sat side-by-side on the sofa.

We sang some of her favorite songs together, and when the other residents heard us singing, they joined in. Carolyn cuddled up to me and smiled the whole time I was there. However, as I got up to leave, she said to me frankly, "You're still too skinny."

When Mary returned from vacation, I let her know how the two visits had progressed. We laughed together about Carolyn mixing us up. The following day, after Mary had gone to see Carolyn, she phoned to tell me what happened. Apparently, as Mary entered the home and walked up to her, Carolyn made the comment, "Well, now you've gone and gotten too fat!"

That's where Carolyn's story ends for me. I'm not sure how it ended for her.

Case #21

NOBODY HOME

My next assigned case was a woman who re-sided in a local nursing home due to weakness and inability to care for herself. She had no living family, only one dear friend who had been given power of attorney.

When I arrived at the facility, I noted that the patient, Diane, shared a small stark cheer-less room with another woman of the same first name. I wondered if staff ever got them mixed up. Hospice patient Diane was lying in the bed closest to the door. She looked very, very thin and debili-tated. I had been briefed that she suffered from colon cancer, which had metastasized to the bone. I learned that she was six years older than me, far too young in my estimation for a situation or place like this.

When Diane and I met, we instantly liked one

another. She spoke kindly of her hospice experience thus far. She seemed glad that I'd be visiting as she wanted to "make a new friend." She confided that she wanted to get out of the present facility and into a better one; in fact, she'd really "rather go home" which, of course, wasn't possible. This particular nursing home was dismal and the only privacy Diane had was a curtain which, when drawn, separated the two beds. It certainly didn't shut out the noise of the roommate's annoying television, which was at full volume during my visit. I felt frustrated that there was no local inpatient hospice to receive this patient—no place where she could die in a quiet, peaceful setting.

As Diane and I talked, she complained of pain in both shoulders and her left leg. She exhibited pain behaviors, such as rubbing her neck and drawing up her left leg, but she continued to talk in a very intelligent and coherent manner. When I got home, I called my supervisor to tell her of the patient's pain so that the hospice nurse could address the issue.

I visited Diane the following day, a Friday. She had two other visitors when I arrived—her dear friend with the power of attorney and a church member. It was a busy day for Diane as the hospice aide arrived to give her a bath just as the two visitors left. I walked around the facility to give them some privacy. Once the aide left, Diane and

I had a chance to talk. She said her pain medication had been adjusted, and she only had a slight pain in her neck area. She mentioned being fond of the facility's male on-duty nurse who had been very kind to her. In the morning when she told him that the night staff had let her bag (I wasn't sure if she meant her colostomy bag or her urine bag) overflow despite "pushing the call button a 100 times," he said he'd notify the night supervisor so it wouldn't happen again. He had seemed very concerned, which had comforted Diane.

Our next visit was lovely. Diane's roommate had gone to physical therapy so the television was off, which meant Diane and I could share quiet time alone together. She shared various childhood memories with me, including an interesting Halloween adventure in which she and her friend had trick-or-treated at a house owned by actor Bob Cummings, who had opened the door himself. Both girls had been 11 years old at the time and had swooned over meeting this famous celebrity. Diane's story then switched to the present time as she lovingly described three little neighbor children who had worn adorable Halloween costumes when they visited her house this past October. She said she had given them "very special candy bars."

My next visit was on a Monday. Although Diane seemed drowsy from medications, she kept up her end of the conversation. When I admired the crayoned drawings that hung on the wall, Diane said the three little neighbor children had made them for her. She said she had never had children of her own but that the neighbor lady had complemented her on her "natural mothering skills." Diane then despondently referred to the five cats she had given up when she entered the nursing home. To lighten the mood, I asked if she wanted me to bring music with me on my next visit, but she said hearing music made her sad. So, we talked about the many hospice services that were available to her, and she said she'd like to see the hospice chaplain if she could be given a 24-hour notice before the chaplain visited. I reported her request to my supervisor later that day.

The following day when I returned to the nursing home, Diane had some word confusion. She would say a wrong word or not be able to think of a particular word. She'd begin telling a story and then forget what she was saying. Her roommate's TV blared in the background as usual, so I wasn't sure if the problem was from medication or distraction. I had brought a poetry book with me and asked if she'd like me to read from it, but Diane declined, saying she preferred murder mysteries! She then changed topics and told me that her favorite evangelist was Billy Graham, so we talked about him for awhile. Then she looked up at the clock and groaned, saying kitchen staff would soon be bringing a supper tray with food that she didn't want to eat. I noticed that her present tray table had a completely uneaten meal on it as well as two full cartons of juice and a cup of cocoa. She said trying to eat food felt like climbing a mountain. I told her that eating was her choice, and she needn't feel pressured to do so.

I returned two days later and stayed for a half hour. I was surprised to see the drastic change in Diane's condition. She didn't speak or make eye contact. She was unresponsive when I said my name. She lay on her side in a deep sleep with her eyes half open and her mouth agape. She was hooked up to an oxygen machine with a nasal cannula to aid her labored breathing, something she hadn't required previously. The large chair I normally sat in was over on the roommate's side of the room, which meant I had to stand. The roommate was in the other bed with the TV blasting some soap opera replete with yelling and screaming. I wondered if those horrible sounds were being integrated into Diane's dreams. I did notice that someone had given Diane a soft lavender stuffed bunny which was tucked under her left arm. Her eyelids fluttered slightly as I stroked her hair but I didn't say anything as it was impossible to talk over the television.

The next day, I was relieved to find Diane alone in her room. Her roommate's bed was empty although the television was blaring at full volume as always. I immediately turned it off, grateful for the ensuing quiet. Diane looked much the same as she did on my previous visit. She lay on her left side appearing asleep with her eyes half open and her mouth wide open. The oxygen machine droned, although I saw no perceptible rise or fall of her chest. This time, I had brought my camp stool with me so that I could sit next to the side rail and stroke Diane's hair. I told her I was there, although her eyelids did not flutter as I touched her. Diane's forehead and arms felt warm as I lightly caressed her. I spoke quietly about the light she would see when she passed over and how loved ones, such as her parents, would be waiting for her. I told her she'd have a healthy body which would be able to run and dance. I sang hymns softly while watching for any response but saw nothing.

After thirty minutes had elapsed, I checked Diane's nail beds and saw that they were blue. Her hands felt cold to the touch. I noticed she had a rosary clutched in her left hand along with the lavender bunny tucked under that same arm. The other arm cradled a white bunny. Both arms were warm to the touch and neither had any mottling. I pulled the covers up further on her chest to keep her warm. It was hard to tell if she was still alive. I guess I was wondering out loud because I heard myself say, "Diane, are you dead?" There was no response. I decided to give her the benefit of the doubt and moved my stool to the other side of the bed, closer to her face. I continued to stroke her hair for another ten minutes until a nursing home aide popped her head in the doorway to check on Diane. I said I wasn't sure whether or not she was alive. The aide summoned a nurse who confirmed that, indeed, Diane had passed away. The useless oxygen machine was turned off and the nasal cannula removed from her nose. As her body was still warm, the nurse wasn't sure if Diane had passed away before I entered her room or sometime during my visit. Frankly, I'd like to think it happened after I shut off the noisy TV and held her hand.

I told the facility nurse that I had been instructed to call hospice if a patient died in my presence, but I wasn't sure if that meant when it happened in a nursing home setting and, if so, could I use her phone? She said *she'd* call hospice, the funeral home, and the friend who had Diane's power of attorney, as that was *their* policy. The nurse allowed me to remain in the room a few minutes longer with Diane.

I now could see the difference in Diane's eyes from yesterday to today. The previous day, when Diane had been unresponsive and her eyes half-shut, there had been a little gleam directly in the center of her pupils. Today, as I gazed at Diane's droopy eyes, I noticed they were filmy, lightless and lifeless. Now I could see for sure that "nobody was home."

Case #22

THE PATH

When I walked into the room in which this new client was deeply asleep, I sensed that I wasn't there for her, but for her family who hovered near-by. I introduced myself to the patient's daughter, Robin, who was anxiously alternating between sitting and standing. I shook hands with the patient's 19-year-old granddaughter, Mara, who sat cross-legged on the floor next to the bed in obvious distress. I thought about how different this was from my last case. That patient had no family at all.

This particular nursing home was definitely upscale. The patient, Lucy, shared a semi-private room with a bathroom separating the two spacious sections. No one occupied the other bed, which created a welcomed privacy for the family. Lucy's mouth was agape and her breathing ragged but her color looked good and her skin was warm to the touch, including her hands and feet. As she slept, Robin, Mara, and I got to know each other a little better. Robin explained that her mother had only recently been admitted to this facility and to hospice care. Before that, Lucy had lived with Robin's brother in another state; however, when Lucy's health deteriorated, Robin wanted her mother moved nearby. That's when Lucy was brought to this facility.

While we talked, Robin kept repeating that she didn't know why her mother kept hanging on when it was obvious that her body could no longer sustain life. Mara, who had continued to pat her grandmother's hand and remain silent, arose and said she had to go to work. Once she left, Robin shared that Mara was "very close to Lucy" and that she was "taking it hard." Robin and I talked about "unfinished business" and how a patient, despite all physical systems failing, could hang on if they hadn't received closure in a particular area of their life. I mentioned the importance of "quiet time" which can offer an opportunity for a patient to slip away. Robin confessed that she spent most of her waking hours at the facility at her mother's bedside. She felt guilty that she had missed some of Mara's lacrosse try-outs, but she had not wanted to leave her mother alone in the room. We mutually agreed that the following day, Robin would attend one of Mara's lacrosse practices while I stayed with Lucy.

On Saturday, Lucy was alone and asleep when I entered her room. She looked much the same as the previous day. Although she didn't open her eyes, I told her who I was and talked to her about letting go. I quietly sang hymns until Robin and Mara arrived. I spoke to Robin about the possibility of having her brother and sister phone the patient. I suggested that Robin could hold the phone to Lucy's ear so that they could tell her they loved her and encourage her to go to the light and join her husband, who had died several years prior.

On Monday, I visited the patient for over an hour although I didn't spend much time alone with Lucy. The hospice nurse arrived while Robin and I were in the room. After checking Lucy, the nurse said that she remained "status quo." Robin expressed a concern that Lucy had used nine diapers overnight, saying that she had brought in a box of ten the previous evening. When Robin had asked nursing home staff about this problem, she had been told that Lucy "wet a lot." The hospice nurse smiled and said that it was more probable that the diapers Robin brought in had gone to supplement a shortage elsewhere. She suggested writing Lucy's name in permanent marker across the plastic area of the diapers. As Robin had brought in a new package of Depends and I had a black marker in my bag, we sat together and labeled the diapers. It

reminded us both of marking our children's clothing before they went off to camp!

After the hospice nurse left, Robin mentioned
that Mara had just started a new job but would
stop by as soon as she got off work. Robin seemed
concerned that Mara was spending every free
moment with her grandmother, which was deplet-
ing Mara's emotional and physical reserves. I told
Robin that this was my concern also, not only for
Mara but for her.

When Mara did arrive, I asked if she'd be
willing to speak with me privately and she agreed.
The two of us went to a quiet, unpopulated area
of the nursing home to talk about the process of
letting go—how both patient and family had to
find their own way to let go. I shared an intimate
detail of my own hospice training as I wanted to
reach out to this hurting teenager. I told her about
the hospice guided imagery session in which we
had to pretend we were the person dying. The
lights had been dimmed and soft music played in
the background. We were instructed to write the
names of people and places we deeply loved on
ten pieces of paper. We put those beloved items in
an imaginary backpack while we walked along an
imaginary woodland path by a beautiful lake on a
gorgeous day. A bright light shone that beckoned
us and we felt the need to move towards it. We
were instructed that we couldn't ever turn back

but must continue to move forward. As we traveled along this path toward the warm beautiful light, our load became very heavy and we were told to stop along the path to lighten it. Each time we stopped, we had to remove an item from our backpack. I cried at having to leave behind places and people I loved, but I also felt the overwhelming love and warmth that beckoned me forward along this path. As I finished relating the meditation, Mara and I cried together. We hugged and Mara said she had a better understanding of the issues that faced her grandmother and herself

I returned the following Tuesday afternoon to find Robin sitting next to Lucy's bed as usual. I noticed that Lucy's left hand was swollen and had been positioned carefully on a pillow. Her feet and hands felt cold to me and there was a hint of mottling on the back of her big toe. Otherwise, Lucy's color was good and she was sleeping peacefully. Robin seemed emotionally drained and said she had cried most of the day. She related that the previous night she had called her brother and requested that he speak to their mother to urge her to "let go." Robin had held the phone up to Lucy's ear and could hear her brother "tell mom that he loved her" but, before ending the call, he said he hoped she would "rally and get well." This had really upset Robin so I suggested we go to a quiet, out of earshot area to talk privately, which we did.

Mostly, I just listened to her as she needed to vent her anger and verbalize her fears.

When Robin finished talking, I asked if Mara had shared the imaginary spiritual "walk down the path" that she and I had taken the previous day. Robin said no but that Mara seemed in a better place emotionally. Although painful to rehash, I knew I needed to share 'the walk' with Robin, which I did. She told me afterward that she had experienced an "aha" moment. We hugged and agreed that I would return to see Lucy in three days but that never happened.

Early Friday morning, Robin called to say her mother had died gently at 2 a.m. Robin's voice sounded peaceful and resolved. She shared that both she and Mara had spent time the previous afternoon talking to Lucy about the dying process and how getting well again was not an option. Lucy had remained asleep but they had each bent over to talk quietly in her ear. They had told her to "go towards the light and be with daddy." After that, they had both gone home to rest. Although she hadn't been with Lucy when she died, Robin felt she had truly helped her mother finally cross over.

Case #23

UH-HUH

When I was assigned as her Hospice volunteer, Mrs. Mart was 92 years old and resided in an assisted living facility. Her general diagnosis was debility, with secondary problems of urinary tract infections, dehydration, and foot ulcers.

My initial visit found Mrs. Mart living on the first floor of the facility. A large window filled her room with sunlight. A dresser, footstool, floor lamp, lounge chair, and colorful afghan made the room seem like a real home. Physically, Mrs. Mart lay in a hospital bed on her back with her mouth partially open. Her eyelids fluttered when I identified myself as her hospice volunteer. She was generally nonverbal, other than responding positively with an occasional "uh-huh" graced by a smile. Her eyes never opened. Her hands made scratching movements at the top of her nightgown, and she seemed somewhat restless, so I pulled my camp stool close to her bed and asked if it would be all right if I sang to her. She responded with another "uh-huh." I chose some old-time favorite tunes and sang for approximately an hour. To my surprise, she tried to hum along to some of them, such as "Embraceable You," "Red River Valley," "How Great Thou Art," and "America the Beautiful." By the time I left that day, her hands had stopped clutching at her nightgown and her body lay relaxed.

I visited Mrs. Mart again the following day. This time she was lying sound asleep on her side. Her mouth was wide open and she occasionally snored. There was no "uh-huh" when I told her who I was. I sang only the songs she had responded to the previous day, hoping that she'd hum along, but she didn't. I did notice that her level of consciousness seemed to lighten while I sang. Her breathing became less deep, as if she was trying to listen.

Unfortunately, Mrs. Mart died before my next visit. Even as I write about our short time together, I can mentally imagine her saying "uh-huh."

Case #24

BUBBLES

When assigned to this 96-year-old patient, I was impressed by her unusual first name, Royce, only to learn that she wanted to be called by her nickname, Lindy. She had no active disease process other than old age and very poor hearing. Eventually, she was discharged from hospice due to good health!

Lindy resided in the Alzheimer's unit of a local assisted living facility although she did not have dementia at all! I'm still not sure why she was housed in that particular unit. She sat in a wheelchair in the common area along with several other patients when I first visited her. I had brought a sing-along video with me, which I placed into the unit's VCR and, to my surprise, every resident joined in singing. Lindy was the only one, however, who knew all the words to "You Are My Sunshine" and several other songs. After the video was finished, she asked who I was, and I explained that I was a hospice volunteer who would be visiting her frequently. She seemed satisfied with that explanation.

I visited Lindy several times over the next two months. She was able to sit in a wheelchair in the dining room and eat all three meals by herself, much to my amazement. She was thin as a rail but ate like a horse. Sometimes when I arrived, she appeared to be taking a nap. At those times, she would open her eyes and say she was only resting her eyelids for want of anything better to do. We'd sing her favorite songs together at bedside. If I sang a song she didn't know, she'd tap out the beat on the bedrail with her fingers. She had a great sense of rhythm.

On one visit, I brought bubbles with me to release while we sang the song, "I'm Forever Blowing Bubbles." As the bubbles floated around the room, she laughed so loudly that we had to stop singing until she caught her breath. She then insisted that I bring the bubbles with me every time I visited.

As she got to know me better, Lindy talked more freely and openly. She shared many memories of her younger days. There was a warbling quality to her speech, probably due to aged vocal cords. She was very coherent, opinionated, and funny.

After 90 days in our program, regulations required that Lindy be re-evaluated by the hospice nurse. Her condition was upgraded, which was good news to everyone but me, as she was discharged from hospice care. I said a final goodbye to Lindy on our last day together. She called to me loudly as I was leaving the unit, "Drive safely. I love you."

Case #25

A LITTLE LONGER

When I first met Missy, my latest Hospice assignment, I recognized her immediately. She was the lady who would raise one finger of her hand as a greeting whenever I visited another woman on the Alzheimer's Unit of this particular assisted living center.

Missy was eating lunch when I entered the dining room on my initial visit. I had been briefed that she had terminal colon cancer and dementia. Despite that diagnosis, I found her to be very alert and mentally intact. I introduced myself as her hospice volunteer who would visit regularly. She seemed delighted and told me her given name was Maybell, but that she preferred to be called Missy. She told me about her family and medical situation. I was impressed that she could eat by herself and be so coherent.

The second time I visited Missy, it was again at noontime. I expected to find her in the dining room, but she wasn't there. An activities aide said that she thought Missy had refused lunch and asked to lie down, but this wasn't entirely true. When I entered her room, I was greeted by Missy's son and his girlfriend. According to them, they had arrived a half hour earlier and were just as baffled as I was at this change of condition. Missy was now on oxygen and not responding to questions. A social worker from hospice arrived for her regular visit while the three of us were still with Missy. Upon assessing the situation, the social worker put in a call to the hospice nurse.

While we were awaiting the nurse, Missy's son, Brad, filled us in on some family history, including the fact that his brother had died a few years earlier from leukemia. He said his mother had lost her will to live after her youngest son's death. To me, Missy didn't seem a bit like the woman I had met just a few days prior. I left before the hospice nurse arrived.

Missy was still bedridden when I visited three days later. The hospice aide had just finished bathing her when I entered the room. Missy was semi-comatose with labored breathing. Her coloring was good, her hands warm, and her nail beds pink. The aide said Missy's blood pressure was also good and added that she had been with Missy the day of the "food incident." Apparently, Missy had been eating lunch when she appeared to choke on some broccoli. The choking was later attributed to a stroke in progress. At that time, Missy was put on oxygen but never fully regained consciousness. The right side of her body remained paralyzed.

After the aide left, I sang to Missy. There was an occasional opening of her left eye but it seemed vacant. I was only able to spend a few moments alone with Missy before Brad and his girlfriend arrived. Before I left, we talked about Missy's rapid decline since the stroke.

The hospice nurse was with Missy on my next visit. She changed the Scopolamine patch that was behind Missy's ear to help dry up the fluid in her lungs. Brad was also there, and we talked about possible unfinished family business that might be keeping Missy from moving on.

Two days later when I visited, Missy's right eye remained at half mast, and both eyes looked filmy. Her left eye would open occasionally, but she didn't speak. Because we were alone, I turned off the harsh overhead light as well as the droning television, and opened the drapes to allow natural light to cast a soft glow in the room. I put a stuffed animal under her right hand and sang some hymns quietly before leaving.

On a subsequent visit, I sang and held Missy's left hand. I was surprised when I felt a gentle squeeze. On some level, Missy was aware she wasn't alone.

Missy did not squeeze my hand on my next visit. She no longer looked pink. She had been 15 days without food or water. When Brad arrived, we agreed that whenever one of us was with her, we'd encourage Missy to go towards the light and to look for her youngest son who had already made the transition.

I was supposed to visit Missy the following Friday, but I felt compelled to go a day earlier. Missy was alone when I entered her room. I noticed that her hands were cold and bluish. She was panting rather than breathing normally. Her legs were mottled, but the mottling had not yet reached her arms. I sang and prayed aloud, asking Missy to focus on going towards the light and her loved ones. While I was there, the hospice nurse came in to administer a dose of Morphine to help with Missy's heavy panting. The nurse said we were "close," and she phoned Missy's son, who said he'd be there in an hour. The nurse leaned over Missy's ear and told her that Brad was coming. I hoped I might have the privilege of being with Missy when she made her final exit, but a half hour later, I had to leave. Missy was still alive at that time. I kissed her goodbye and told her I'd return the following day.

The phone was ringing when I arrived home

40 minutes later. It was my hospice supervisor advising me that Missy had died! I was temporarily speechless and then told my supervisor that I had just been with Missy, singing hymns, and hoping she would pass on my watch.

Later, the thought struck me that maybe Missy had been wondering when the woman (me) would stop singing and leave the room so she could die in peace! When I shared this thought with my daughter, she said, "Mom, did you ever think that your patient was enjoying the music so much that she decided to stay a little longer?"

EPILOG

In July 2005 when the last client mentioned in *Hospice Journeys* died, I took a break from hospice due to family issues. My single brother, who lived and worked in Florida, was sick, depressed, and had financial problems. My husband and I had urged him to leave Florida and move in with us. Instead, in November of 2005, he took his own life.

Despite my hospice volunteer and bereavement training, nothing prepared me for the loss of my younger brother. I was ripped apart emotionally. The burden of guilt I carried for not rescuing him was overwhelming. I cried incessantly.

Three months after my brother died, I remained in what felt like the depths of Hell. I would still be there had it not been for two amazing women. Each of them understood the pain I was in because both women had lost family members in this same tragic manner. One of the women brought books for me to read that had helped her, and the other consoled me by phone. The most potent words I heard were: "guilt is a form of control." In other words, I was trying to rewrite history. I needed to accept my brother's death and go on with my life because it was what he would want me to do. Each of these women struggled every day with the same challenge. Perhaps it was those words or perhaps it was knowing someone understood my grief, but my burden of guilt lifted that day and gradually, I was able to function again.

The following year when my mother became ill, I flew to Florida to spend two weeks with her. During that time, I arranged for her admission to Hospice of Palm Beach County. With their help, mother was able to die in her own home, cared for by my sister, and surrounded by friends.

May Hospice Journeys everywhere continue in shared love and peace.

DONATION PAGE

Please consider making a donation to your own local hospice facility. Many hospices are non-profits whose donations are tax-deductible to the fullest extent allowed by law.

A contribution to any hospice will be gratefully appreciated and used to provide the best of services to their clients.

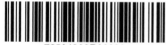

Made in the USA
Middletown, DE
06 May 2018